Learning Disability and Epilepsy: an Integrative Approach

Learning Disability and Epilepsy: an Integrative Approach

Edited by

MICHAEL R. TRIMBLE

*Professor of Behavioural Neurology, Institute of Neurology and
Consultant Physician in Psychological Medicine,
National Hospitals for Neurology and Neurosurgery, London, UK*

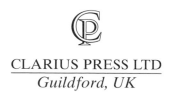

CLARIUS PRESS LTD
Guildford, UK

Published by

Clarius Press Ltd
8 Holly Lea, Guildford,
Surrey GU4 7PG, UK
Tel: +44 (0) 1483 503 206
Fax: +44 (0) 1483 533 928

British Library Cataloguing in Publication Data
A catalogue record for this book is available from the British Library

ISBN   0-9542279-1-3

Composition by Wellset Repro Ltd, Cranleigh, Surrey
Printed and bound in Great Britain by Biddles Ltd, Guildford

Contents

Continued overleaf

Contributors

Richard Appleton, Royal Liverpool Children's NHS Trust, Alder Hey, Eaton Road, Liverpool, UK

Frank M.C. Besag, Bedfordshire and Luton Community NHS Trust, University of Luton, Luton, UK

Tim Betts, Birmingham University Seizure Clinic, Queen Elizabeth Psychiatric Hospital, Birmingham, UK

Stephen W. Brown, Peninsula Medical School, Plymouth, UK

Katie Gould, Birmingham University Seizure Clinic, Queen Elizabeth Psychiatric Hospital, Birmingham, UK

Lyn Greenhill, Birmingham University Seizure Clinic, Queen Elizabeth Psychiatric Hospital, Birmingham, UK

Heather Gregory, The Grovehill Centre, Beverley, Yorkshire, UK

Mike Kerr, University of Wales College of Medicine, Cardiff, UK

Ennapadam S. Krishnamoorthy, Raymond Way Neuropsychiatry Research Group, Institute of Neurology, National Hospital for Neurology and Neurosurgery, Queen Square, London, UK

Jaana Lähdetie, Department of Medical Genetics, Turku University, Turku, Finland

Matti Sillanpää, Department of Child Neurology and Public Health, Turku University, Turku, Finland

Sanjay M. Sisodiya, Department of Clinical and Experimental Epilepsy, Institute of Neurology, National Hospital for Neurology and Neurosurgery, Queen Square, London, UK

Ekkehart F.A. Staufenberg, Norwich Epilepsy Clinic, Department of Neurology, Norfolk and Norwich University Hospital NHS Trust, Norwich, Norfolk, UK

Michael R. Trimble, Institute of Neurology, National Hospital for Neurology and Neurosurgery, Queen Square, London, UK

Preface

Managing people with learning disability is a challenge in its own right, but when learning disability and epilepsy coincide both diagnostic and treatment issues become magnified. It is clear that many people with learning disability, particularly those with more severe disorders, have identifiable neurological impairments, although their management rarely falls squarely with neurologists. Indeed, such are the complexities of clinical presentation that a multidisciplinary approach is required, but often such a team does not incorporate anyone with particular expertise in epilepsy. This is strange as we know that a very high proportion of people with learning disability have epilepsy syndromes and that many people with seizure disorders have learning disability of varying degrees.

Learning disability, in common with other fields of medical practice, has received a considerable boost from recent advances in the underlying scientific basis of medicine. In particular, the use of new imaging techniques to view abnormalities of brain structure and function, the introduction to new genetic understanding and the development of new drugs to help symptoms have all been part of this enterprise.

Further, the adoption of multidisciplinary care programmes has allowed for a much better integrated and coordinated management of learning disability and has facilitated the introduction of specialised services including, for example, developing the role of the epilepsy specialist nurse for people with learning disability.

This book aims to provide an update of scientific and medical knowledge in this area, as well as an insight into how this is contributing to management of patients with these complex problems.

In chapter one the difficult area of definition is discussed, outlining some of the historical principles and the present situation. This is followed by a discussion of the neuroepidemiological aspects of learning disability with specific reference to epilepsy.

The third chapter updates genetics, and this is followed by a chapter that outlines a number of specific epilepsy syndromes that are related to learning disability. The fifth chapter reveals the importance of brain imaging and the discovery of malformations and dysplasias, which are not only very relevant clinically, but also have links to underlying genetic problems.

There then follows a chapter examining associations between learning disability, epilepsy and autism. Much of the converging evidence has to do with possible abnormalities of limbic structures, particularly the amygdala.

Other individual chapters examine the relevance of EEG monitoring in patients, and the importance of uncovering state-dependent learning disabilities. The fascinating ictally-related behavioural syndromes that are in fact inter-ictal, such as post-ictal psychosis and forced normalisation, are also discussed.

Three chapters relate to treatment: the first to anti-epileptic drug therapies with specific reference to patients with learning disability, the second to the evaluation and use of psychotropic drugs in this patient group, and the third to a discussion of environmental and behavioural interventions that are so important for this patient group. Finally, but very importantly, the role of the epilepsy specialist nurse is explored in some detail.

It is hoped that this book will provide for the interested reader an update covering the wide spectrum of topics in the area of learning disability and epilepsy. It also coincides with a growing interest in the relationship between these two spectra of disorders, which should further the management of patients with these problems and lead hopefully to improved quality of life. If exploring some of the underlying scientific developments in this field not only excites the interest of researchers, but also helps to destigmatise people with learning disability, then this will be an additional benefit.

M R TRIMBLE
Institute of Neurology, Queen Square, London
July 2003

1

Towards Definitions: Learning Disability, Mental Handicap and Intelligence

STEPHEN W. BROWN

Peninsula Medical School, Plymouth, UK

'*Feeble-mindedness is hereditary and transmitted as surely as any other character. We cannot successfully cope with these conditions until we recognise feeble-mindedness and its hereditary nature, recognise it early, and take care of it... In considering the question of care, segregation through colonisation seems in the present state of our knowledge to be the ideal and perfectly satisfactory method. Sterilisation may be accepted as a makeshift, as a help to solve this problem because the conditions have become so intolerable. But this must at present be regarded only as a makeshift and temporary, for before it can be extensively practised, a great deal must be learned about the effects of the operation and about the laws of human inheritance*' (Goddard, 1912).

'*Wherever sympathetic magic occurs in its pure unadulterated form, it assumed that in nature one event follows another necessarily and invariably without the intervention of any spiritual or personal agency. Thus its fundamental conception is identical with that of modern science; underlying the whole system is a faith, implicit but real and firm, in the order and uniformity of nature*' (Frazer, 1900).

INTRODUCTION

This chapter will attempt to trace the origins of current concepts of developmental or intellectual disabilities and how these came to be viewed as separate from insanity, with a consideration of the attempts at measurement and classification.

In the search for acceptable phraseology a number of terms have been used in different countries and at different times. These differences continue to cause misunderstanding not least in the scientific community. It is important that those working in the field, whether as clinicians or researchers, have an understanding of the range of nomenclature and definitions, so that appropriate conclusions can be drawn from research.

Since epilepsy and its treatment may be associated with cognitive impairments that can range from severe to none at all, which can be global or discrete, and which can be permanent or intermittent, a bewildering range of possible descriptions is available. People may be variously described as having 'disabilities', 'difficulties' or a 'deficiency', or as being 'retarded' or 'handicapped', and these problems may have been regarded as arising in 'developmental', 'intellectual' or just plain 'mental' spheres.

The term 'learning disability' is used today in the United Kingdom to describe an area that is elsewhere called 'mental retardation'. However in North America, discrete impairments of certain cognitive functions in children without mental retardation are referred to as 'learning disabilities'. For example, in one standard textbook aimed mainly at the United States market, a chapter entitled *'Mental Retardation'* covers the area familiar to learning disability specialists in the United Kingdom, but is immediately followed by two chapters on *'Dyslexia and other Language-Based Learning Disabilities'* and *'Nonverbal Learning Disabilities and Motor Skills Disorders'*, neither of which would be recognised as covering the specialty by colleagues on the other side of the Atlantic Ocean (Coffey and Brumback, 1998). Other terms used internationally include those that translate as 'mental handicap' (France, Flemish-speaking Belgium and, until relatively recently, United Kingdom), 'intellectual disability' (Japan and Australia) and 'developmental disability' (Canada).

There is often a difference between everyday usage and professional terminology. In Italy and in Israel the general population may refer to people being 'mentally retarded', while professionals refer to 'intellectual disabilities', and 'developmental disabilities' respectively. The people for whom these terms were devised, for example those represented by the international group 'People First', do not always take the same view as their physicians or psychologists. People First in the United Kingdom has indicated that a preferred term might be 'learning difficulty'. This term is also used by educationalists to describe discrete types of learning problems such as dyslexia, but nevertheless some services that were formerly named as Learning Disability Services have changed their names to reflect this.

HISTORY

Most human cultures seem to make provision for people who lack the capacity to be responsible for their actions. In ancient Hebrew law, idiots, lunatics, and children below a certain age were not held criminally responsible, because they could not distinguish good from evil or right from wrong, and were thus considered blameless. The wording of the law is interesting, partly because there is an implied distinction between idiocy and madness on one hand, but also because there is an implied developmental view – small children lack this capacity but under normal circumstances would acquire it at a certain age. Some people might not so develop and thus become idiots; while in other cases (madness) the defect of reasoning is acquired.

In countries whose legal systems derive from Anglo-Saxon or British traditions, the English King Edward II is generally credited with making the first legal distinction between idiocy and insanity. In 1307, the statute *De Prerogativa Regis* distinguished, for the purposes of property rights, between those who were incompetent due to being born fools from those whose abilities might recover. The capacity test used at that time was whether or not the person's mental ability was more or less than that of a 'wild beast'.

After the time of Edward II, although idiocy and insanity were distinguished, there was a tendency to class idiocy and dementia together. These terms were separated in nineteenth century European thought, when views were also taken on possible causes. A minority view, offered by Pinel, was that 'excessive intemperance and venery' could cause idiocy, and others thought masturbation was a factor, while the celebrated physician J.L.H. Down hypothesised that it was a possible outcome if the father was drunk when the child was conceived (Miller, 1995). Other associations that were promoted as relevant included the shape of the palate. Down regarded palatal deformity as a universal feature of idiocy, although he later stated that this only applied to 'genetous' (congenital) cases (Down, 1862). In rebuttal, Shaw (1876) studied large numbers of subjects and found no association between high-arched palate and idiocy.

A received view in the mid-nineteenth century was that that idiocy resulted from a lack of sensory input, and that therefore it might be correctable by teaching. The English Commissioners in Lunacy reported in 1865 that,

'The benefits to be derived, even in idiot cases apparently hopeless… from persevering endeavours to develop the dormant powers, physical and intellectual, are now so fully established, that any argument on the subject would be superfluous' (Miller, 1995).

This optimistic humanism spawned various methods of remediation, including Seguin's emphasis on training sensory and motor functioning, and Guggenbuhl's work in a Swiss centre caring for children with cretinism.

He emphasised good diet, baths, physical exercise and special training procedures for the sensory systems. These holistic and humanistic approaches
might be echoed in modern times by movements such as conductive education or mediated learning (Cottam and Sutton, 1999; Feuerstein *et al.*, 1988)
although they have not suffered the same fate. Unfortunately for
Guggenbuhl's work, however, subsequent investigation rebutted his claims
and the method fell into disrepute (Miller, 1995).

As this happened another, darker concept emerged and took intellectual
hold; the theory of degeneracy. As propounded by B.A.Morel (1857) this
linked insanity, criminality, epilepsy, dementia and idiocy in a grand unifying
scheme held together with theologically derived pseudogenetics. Morel, and
those of the degeneracy school, proposed that although mental disorders
might have an external or environmental cause in the first instance, the
person's biological state is then modified, so that the disorder becomes
hereditary. Following this, each generation displays an increasing degree of
pathology until the line becomes extinguished in idiocy. Although degeneration was exemplified by the deterioration across generations, it could also
take place within the person's lifetime. Some writers saw degeneration as
analogous, and possibly homologous, with the fall of man from the Garden of
Eden. Morel also had a particular interest in epilepsy, and was responsible for
suggesting that there could exist a masked form, *'epilepsie larvée'*, in which
the main features were not seizures but insanity. During the second half of
the nineteenth century many European medical writers took this as received
fact.

In the United Kingdom one of the most significant expressions of degeneracy theory was Down's description of the syndrome that bears his name
(Down, 1866). He noted *'I have for some time ... had my attention directed to
the possibility of making a classification of the feeble-minded, by arranging
them around various ethnic standards... I have been able to find among the
large number of idiots and imbeciles which come under my observations...
that a considerate portion can be fairly referred to one of the great divisions of
the human family other than the class from which they have sprung'* (Down,
1866).

Down was able to divide many of his patients up into Malays, Ethiopians,
Red Indians and Mongolians. He thought Mongolism was *'for the most part,
instances of degeneracy arising from tuberculosis in the parents'*. To Down,
Europeans obviously represented the summit of creation, but the exhibition
of characteristics of inferior racial types could occur as a consequence of
impaired or arrested development. Therefore Mongolism represented degeneration to a more primitive type.

Although degeneracy theory officially faded from fashion by the beginning
of the twentieth century, it was part of the shadowy origins of eugenics, and
eugenics, together with the parallel emerging disciplines of anthropometry

and psychometry, gave birth to modern theories and practices of IQ testing and concepts of retardation and learning disability.

Idiots, imbeciles, morons and eugenics

The term 'idiot' has been used since medieval times. Idiocy was apparently viewed as a unitary condition, and its description and classification were based on its severity. Some people although obviously affected by the underlying condition, were less incapable than others, even though they were still unable to live independently. These came to be called 'imbeciles'. At the beginning of the twentieth century, Goddard, riding the crest of the wave of eugenics, coined the term 'moron' from the Greek *moros* (foolish). Morons, or high-grade feeble-minded people might look normal, and, unlike true idiots, they were likely to procreate, so that their feeble-mindedness would be passed on to their offspring. Their lack of ability to learn and their simple minds meant that they were vulnerable to becoming criminals, and their fecundity and ability to be easily led into immoral ways meant that there was a danger of society becoming overwhelmed.

'We have come to the point where we no longer leave babies or little children to die uncared for in our streets, but who has yet thought of caring intelligently for the vastly more pathetic child-man or child-woman, who through matured sex powers, which they do not understand, fill our land with its overflowing measure of misery and crime?...... The idiot is not our greatest problem. He is indeed loathsome; he is somewhat difficult to take care of; nevertheless, he lives his life and is done. He does not continue the race with a line of children like himself. Because of his very low-grade condition, he never becomes a parent. It is the moron type that makes for us our great problem. And ... we face the question, "What is to be done with them..." (Goddard, 1912).

Goddard considered euthanasia as an option, but thought it might not be acceptable to the public, so he cautiously raised the possibility of sterilisation to stop society as a whole being dragged down by the burden of accommodating increasing numbers of the feeble-minded. Similar arguments were heard 30 years later in Germany. Goddard's book was first published in Germany in 1914, and enjoyed a substantial reprint in 1933 after the Nazis came to power. In 1906 Goddard became the first director of the Vineland Psychological Research Laboratory in New Jersey, linked to the New Jersey Training School for the feebleminded, which had been founded in 1888. The Vineland name lives on in test scales used today to assess people with developmental disabilities, the Vineland Adaptive Behavior Scales or VABS (Sparrow *et al.*, 1984). The use of the VABS in research situations frequently also requires a statistical process associated with another name linked to the eugenic movement, Karl Pearson.

Reading such historical narratives in modern textbooks might seduce us into believing that there was an intellectual consensus in the past, and that ideas developed and evolved in some way which, when we look back, reflect a logical progression. In fact, narrative is an attempt to impose such a view, by taking examples from those writings that survive, often in English or with a European perspective. It is difficult to comment on what lay (or non literary or non intellectual) views were in the past, and it may be that there was a greater richness and diversity of opinion than is realized.

ANTHROPOMETRY, PSYCHOMETRY AND IQ

In 19th century London, Sir Francis Galton's 'Anthropometric Laboratory' in South Kensington allowed visitors to pay to have exact measurements made of their height, weight, breathing power, strength of pull and squeeze, colour sense and much else. Galton (1822-1911) was a gentleman-scholar, explorer, meteorologist and cousin of Charles Darwin. He was also interested in explaining the differences between individuals and became convinced that heredity was of prime importance in defining them. His protégé Karl Pearson (1857-1936) occupied the post of Galton Professor of Eugenics at University College London after Galton died. Both Galton and Pearson believed that human abilities followed a normal distribution that could be represented by a bell-shaped curve, and these views were to be influential in the subsequent design of Intelligence Quotient (IQ) tests.

In 1905 Binet and Simon published a 'measuring scale of intelligence' to identify children who might need special education (Binet and Simon, 1905). Some of the tests had precursors in the nineteenth century (including digit span, previously used in Galton's laboratory), and some were new. Although some items were concerned with visuo-motor skill, there was an emphasis on linguistic ability, which caused criticism later. The scale was administered and scored by assigning each test to an age level at which most children performed it successfully, and the child was tested by finding the age level at which most tests were failed. This gave a quantifiable measure of 'mental age', which could be compared to the child's chronological age. Within a short time Binet and Simon's scale was translated into other languages, and, with time, adaptations for an adult population were produced. One of the most enthusiastic advocates of this new intelligence testing was Goddard, who used it in the Kallikak studies referred to earlier (Goddard, 1912).

Binet's system, born of humanitarian desire to identify children in need of special education, used the concept of mental age that was probably reasonable for its time and purpose. Such a concept may be inappropriate for adult populations, and most psychologists would agree it is less helpful today.

Nevertheless, it seems to remain beloved of legal authorities, even though perhaps the time has come to lay it to rest.

Today the most widely used psychometric tests that purport to measure intelligence are the various Wechsler scales. There have been four versions of the adult scales. The first of these, the Wechsler-Bellevue Intelligence Scale was published in 1939. The Wechsler Adult Intelligence Scale (WAIS) followed this in 1955. The WAIS was revised and re-standardised in 1981 (WAIS-R) and revised and standardised again in 1997 (WAIS-III). These revisions have implications for long-term monitoring of cognitive abilities both in individuals and in populations, as will be discussed below.

David Wechsler had the idea to develop a new scale when working as a US Army psychologist at the end of the First World War. He noticed that measurements of mental ability on recruits mainly using tests that originated from Binet and seemed to underestimate people's abilities. He attributed this to Binet's tests having an undue emphasis on verbal skill acquisition through formal education. Wechsler then worked with Spearman and Pearson in London before eventually in 1932 becoming chief psychologist at Bellevue Psychiatric Hospital in New York. By 1939 he had developed a new test battery, mainly containing older tests, that should be taken as a whole, but which were subdivided into verbal and non-verbal items. Until then Intelligence Quotient (IQ) was defined in terms of mental age (calculated from the formula: mental age divided by chronological age and multiplied by 100). Wechsler changed the concept of IQ from the mental age-chronological age ratio to one based on a standard score with the same distribution at each age level. Later, Wechsler's approach was extended to children's tests with the Wechsler Intelligence Scale for Children (WISC) and the Wechsler Preschool and Primary Scale of Intelligence (WPPSI). Thus the Binet and Simon test, which had been developed originally in children, had been extended to adults, while Wechsler's test for adults was used as a basis for constructing new scales for children. These days, in test interpretation, in contrast to Wechsler's original intention, there is much emphasis on considering the different subtests as if they are separate measures of specific abilities rather than different approaches to an overarching general intelligence. The WAIS was also not originally intended for assessing people with brain damage, yet it has found use in this area (Boake, 2002).

Implications of different revisions of the WAIS

By definition IQ scores in the general population should follow a bell-shaped normal distribution curve, and the mean IQ score of the population is 100. If, as years pass, the population seems to get better at doing the tests, then even though the 'intelligence' of the population might be increasing (if that is what IQ tests measure), the criteria for scoring the tests need adjusting to bring IQ back into line. The last revision of the WAIS in 1997 raised some issues about the interpretation of discrepancies between the 1997 and 1981 versions. This is discussed by Tulsky and Ledbetter (2000), who emphasise differences in interpreting score discrepancies between the two versions if the clinician switches from WAIS-R to WAIS-III. They point out that *'For IQ tests it becomes imperative that new normative information on the scales is collected every 10 to 15 years so that the average IQ score can be "re-anchored" at 100.'*

Flynn (1984) calculated that the average Full Scale IQ would be increasing by one third to half a point every year. The implication of this is that over a 50 year period, the IQ of the population will actually rise by between 16-25 points, but this is hidden by re-standardising the tests to bring the mean back to a score of 100. The reasons for the rise are presumably related to improvements in education, nutrition and medical care, and speculating about them is beyond the scope of this chapter.

However, mental retardation or intellectual / developmental / learning disability is partly defined and diagnosed by using IQ tests. One of the planks of diagnosis is often taken to be an IQ of 70 or less. The diagnostic concepts have been present since IQ tests were developed. Perhaps we should therefore ponder that an IQ of 70 on the WAIS-III of 1997 is actually equivalent at least to an IQ of between 86 and 95 on the Wechsler-Bellevue test of 1939. The population of people who might be defined as having mental retardation or developmental / intellectual / learning disability might be the same proportion of the overall population as before, because of the statistical nature of the definition, but if IQ tests measure anything worthwhile, it means that this group's needs and abilities fall in a narrower range than previously.

But what do IQ test measure? Is this the same as intelligence? Wechsler (1974) once referred to it as *'the overall capacity of an individual to understand and cope with the world around him.'* At least four concepts are currently in fashion; Spearman's 'g', Sternberg's three sub-theories, Gardner's seven types plus experience, and Horn's fluids & crystals. Each is now considered in turn.

'g' – General ability to deal with cognitive complexity

A concept first advocated by Spearman (1904), 'g' is considered by some to be the main thing that IQ tests measure, and supporters might argue against over-interpretation of subtest scores while looking at the general picture from the total score. Overall IQ had been shown to correlate with a variety of physiological measures including reaction time, speed of processing, brain energy utilisation (higher IQ people use less energy than lower IQ people doing the same task) and (less strongly), brain size, after adjusting for height, weight and gender. These findings are used to justify the notion that for practical purposes intelligence is an innate and generalised function with a physiological substrate (Gottfredson, 1997).

J.C.Raven published a test specifically developed from Spearman's theory in 1938, which involved progressively difficult non-verbal tasks involving choosing the missing component of a matrix pattern from a selection. Raven's Progressive Matrices now exist in a number of formats. The tests are easy to administer, relatively uncontaminated by linguistic background, and often used today as alternatives to the WAIS, especially when balanced in combination with other more specifically verbal tests (Raven, 1960).

Other theories stress what might be called the internal structure of intelligence, and are sometimes referred to as multiple intelligences.

Sternberg's three sub-theories

Robert Sternberg (1985) outlined what he called a triarchic theory of intelligence, consisting of three sub-theories or dimensions (Sternberg, 1985). The *Analytic* or *Componential Dimension* is concerned with structures and mechanisms that underlie the ability to control and monitor processing, execute plans and encode and assemble new knowledge. The *Practical* or *Contextual Dimension* is concerned with the ability to adapt to or reshape the environment, recognising that intelligent behaviour is defined by the socio-cultural context in which it takes place. Thirdly the *Creative* or *Experiential Dimension* addresses the relationship between behaviour in a given situation and the individual's previous amount of experience in that situation. Sternberg proposes that the interaction of all three sub-theories is necessary for a complete explanation of intelligence.

The triarchic theory differs from other theories in its attempts to include both practical and creative intellectual activities. Sternberg believes that standard IQ tests are flawed because they fail adequately to address cultural discrepancies, which in his theory are covered in the contextual dimension. Sternberg has been working on developing his own test, the Sternberg Triarchic Abilities Test or STAT (Sternberg *et al.*, 2001). Sternberg is also well-known for his Triangular Theory of Love (Sternberg, 1998).

Gardner's seven types plus experience

Howard Gardner has suggested that there are at least seven relatively independent types of intelligence, which he lists as logical-mathematical, linguistic, musical, spatial, bodily-kinesthetic, interpersonal, and intrapersonal. Each of these will be modified in its expression by experience. IQ tests are therefore criticised for reducing intelligence to a single test score, and a profiling approach is advocated.

Sternberg and Gardner therefore stand in opposition to the proponents of 'g'.

Horn: fluid & crystallised intelligence

Horn's theory considers intelligence to be built from two broad factors supported by various specific factors. The two broad factors are concerned with what he calls fluid abilities and crystallised abilities. *Fluid intelligence* represents problem solving and reasoning ability when presented with unfamiliar situations. It is tapped by performance subtests of the WAIS, and possibly peaks in adulthood and may decline with age. *Crystallised intelligence* is consequent on the extent to which knowledge of the culture has been attained. Most of the verbal subtests of the WAIS are concerned with it, and it may be relatively resistant to decline as part of ageing.

Many researchers have found Horn's concepts valuable, and at the present time the fluid and crystalline theories seem to be gaining ground.

CLASSIFICATIONS AND DEFINITIONS

Table 1.   Some codes from ICD6 (1948).

325	*Mental deficiency*
325.0	Idiocy
325.1	Imbecility
325.2	Moron
325.3	Borderline intelligence
325.4	Mongolism
325.5	Other and unspecified types
326	*Other and unspecified character, behaviour and intelligence disorders*
326.0	Specific learning defects
326.1	Stammering and stuttering of non-organic origin
326.2	Other speech impediments of non-organic origin
326.3	Acute situational maladjustment
326.4	Other and unspecified

The current Tenth Revision of the International Statistical Classification of Diseases and Related Health Problems, known as ICD10 (World Health Organisation, 1992) is the latest in a series that was formalized in 1893 as the Bertillon Classification or International List of Causes of Death. In the second revision published in 1909 there is a code for idiocy and imbecility, and another for cretinism. In 1938 with the 5th revision, the term changed to mental deficiency, and with the 6th revision in 1948 mental deficiency was broken down into subtypes, while some other specific learning problems were also included. The list from ICD6 is shown in Table 1. The equivalent list from the current ICD10 is shown in Table 2 where the term 'mental retardation' is used.

The ICD10 criteria for diagnosing mental retardation are based on two main components, low cognitive ability and diminished social competence characterised by impairment of skills manifested during the developmental period. IQ is used to define the four categories of severity (Table 3). If IQ alone were used, about 3% of the population would be regarded as qualifying, since the tests are constructed so that about 97% will score 70 or more.

Table 2.   Categories in ICD10

(F70-F79)	*Mental retardation*
F70	Mild mental retardation
F71	Moderate mental retardation
F72	Severe mental retardation
F73	Profound mental retardation
F78	Other mental retardation
F79	Unspecified mental retardation
(F80-F89)	*Disorders of psychological development*
F80	Specific developmental disorders of speech and language
F80.0	Specific speech articulation disorder
F80.1	Expressive language disorder
F80.2	Receptive language disorder
F80.3	Acquired aphasia with epilepsy [Landau-Kleffner]
F80.8	Other developmental disorders of speech and language
F80.9	Developmental disorder of speech and language, unspecified
F81	Specific developmental disorders of scholastic skills
F81.0	Specific reading disorder
F81.1	Specific spelling disorder
F81.2	Specific disorder of arithmetical skills
F81.3	Mixed disorder of scholastic skills
F81.8	Other developmental disorders of scholastic skills
F81.9	Developmental disorder of scholastic skills, unspecified

Table 3.   ICD10 categories for mental retardation defined by IQ

	Category	IQ
F70	Mild	50-69
F71	Moderate	35-49
F72	Severe	20-34
F73	Profound	<20

a fourth character may be added to specify the extent of behavioural impairment:

F7x.0	No or minimal impairment of behaviour
F7x.1	Significant impairment requiring attention or treatment
F7x.8	Other impairments of behaviour
F7x.9	Without mention of impairment of behaviour

The main alternative classification system currently in use is DSM-IV-TR (American Psychiatric Association, 2000), and this uses substantially the same criteria but is more precise. Thus three criteria must be fulfilled: significantly sub-average intellectual functioning (e.g. IQ of < 70), certain defects in adaptive functioning and onset before age 18. For the second criterion, there must be significant limitations in adaptive functioning in at least two of the following domains: communication, self-care, domestic skills, social skills, self-direction, community academic skills, work, leisure, and health and safety.

Another similar definition comes from the American Association on Mental Retardation, the AAMR, (which has recently proposed a name change to the American Association on Intellectual Disabilities or AAID). The AAMR published a new definition of mental retardation, describing it as *'a disability characterised by significant limitations both in intellectual functioning and in adaptive behavior as expressed in conceptual, social, and practical adaptive skills. This disability originates before age 18'* (American Association on Mental Retardation, 2002).

Many workers have felt that the above definitions are insufficient to describe the nature of the problems that users of services face. The World Health Organisation developed a tool for classifying the consequences of diseases, formerly referred to as the International Classification of Impairments, Disabilities and Handicap, but in its most recent revision known as the International Classification of Functioning, Disability and Health, or ICF (World Health Organisation, 2001a). This aims to provide a standard language and framework for the description of health states, and is based on dimensions of functioning with categories, or domains, within each dimension. These dimensions are (1) body functions and structure, (2) activities at the individual level and (3) participation in society. It systematically groups different health domains and health-related domains (e.g. what a person can do or does do when he or she has a given health condition). The health domains are described at body, individual and society dimensions. Although this may be useful in research and in comparing data between countries, the checklist runs to 14 pages (World Health Organisation, 2001b) and its clinical utility may be limited.

SOME OTHER CONCEPTS

Developmental psychology has been highly influenced by the notion of unfolding cognitive schemata described by Piaget and elaborated with regard to mental retardation by Inhelder (1968). She suggested that degrees of retardation coincided with arrest at different stages in Piaget's developmental theory. Thus the subcategories of mental retardation of the ICD10 coincide with developmental arrest at the different Piagetian stages, with profound retardation roughly approximating to Piaget's sensorimotor level, severe retardation to early preoperational stage, moderate retardation to later preoperational levels and mild retardation to the concrete operational stage. This in some ways looks back to Binet. Attempts at including Piagetian tasks into tests have not resulted in enthusiastic uptake, and although Piaget's wider notion of underlying structures in cognitive development still has some support, modern writers stress the importance of flexibility and interaction (Harris, 1995).

The ICD10 and DSM-IV now recognise a variety of other learning disorders that are distinct from mental retardation. The most common of these is dyslexia, but others include specific problems with spelling, written expression and various motor skills disorders. There is an implication that such disorders can exist in isolation from each other, although this is not always the case. There are also a number of other conditions that can affect learning and cognitive ability or which may be associated with educational difficulties, including the DSM concept of attention deficit / hyperactivity disorder, and the pervasive developmental disorders or autistic spectrum disorders. It is uncommon to find these in isolation, and the overlap causes some confusion, yet the problem lies in the classification system. Gillberg has suggested an overarching category of deficits in attention, motor control and perception, or DAMP, and has continued to follow up children with DAMP into adulthood (Gillberg, 1995). Many children (and adults) with DAMP also have epilepsy. Some degree of learning difficulty is always present, but may not readily fall into the categories on offer in DSM or ICD for mental retardation.

Children (and indeed adults) with epilepsy may experience fluctuating cognitive problems as their ability to attend to their surroundings is influenced by seizures, interictal epileptiform EEG discharges, or possibly antiepileptic drug treatment. These same factors also influence behaviour. The distinction between these temporary and the more permanent learning problems, their relationship to behaviour problems and the overall management strategies that should be adopted are reviewed by Besag (2002 and Chapter 7).

CONCLUSIONS

Concepts of mental retardation have tended to reflect other obsessions that exist in society at the time. The Victorian interest in measurement allowed tests to be developed that served to confirm previous assumptions, and these have become self-perpetuating. Why should we use any definitions at all? These days we might cite the need to offer legal protection from exploitation, the need to identify people who need support, and the need to identify children who would benefit from special education. We might, however, draw a veil over the topic of eugenics, although in the nineteenth century these different strands were essentially all linked. The concept of retardation has been subject to many changes of nomenclature, for political and for advocacy reasons, and will continue to do so, as long as the people that it applies to are on the margins of society.

We should not let our concern with using the right words mask another issue, namely do we still need the concept? We recognise some specific syndromes are linked to clinical presentations that guide us to clinical management. These are often more useful than blanket categories of retardation. Yet there is also overlap between many conditions, which sometimes renders the Jesuitical distinctions necessary for diagnosis to be mainly of intellectual interest. Pragmatically it would seem better to continue to seek ways of assessing people's needs individually in order to try and meet them. Traditional tests may have some heuristic value in this enterprise, even though by using them we continue to perpetuate possibly mythical concepts like global intelligence. Not everyone would agree, of course.

REFERENCES

American Association on Mental Retardation. (2002). *Mental Retardation: Definition, Classification, and Systems of Supports,* 10th edition. Washington, DC.

American Psychiatric Association. (2000). *Diagnostic and Statistical Manual of Mental Disorders,* 4th edition (text revision). Washington, DC.

Besag, F.M. (2002). Childhood epilepsy in relation to mental handicap and behavioural disorders. *J Child Psychol Psychiatry* **43**, 103-131.

Binet, A. and Simon, T. (1905). Méthodes nouvelles pour le diagnostic du niveau intellectual des anormaux. *L'Année Psychologique* **11**, 191-244.

Boake, C. (2002). From the Binet-Simon to the Wechsler-Bellevue: tracing the history of intelligence testing. *J Clin Exp Neuropsychol* **24**, 383-405.

Coffey, C.E., and Brumback, R.A. (1998). *Textbook of Pediatric Neuropsychiatry.* American Psychiatric Press Inc, Washington DC.

Cottam, P.J., and Sutton, A. (1999) (Eds). *Conductive Education: A System for Overcoming Motor Disorder.* Chapman and Hall, London.

Down, J.L.H. (1862). On the condition of the mouth in idiocy. *Lancet* **1**, 186.

Down, J.L.H. (1866). *Observations on an ethnic classification of idiots.* London Hospital Reports, **3**, 259-262.

Feuerstein, R., Rand, Y. and Rynders, J.E. (1988). *Don't Accept Me as I Am: Helping Retarded People to Excel.* Perseus Books, Cambridge, MA.

Flynn, J.R. (1984). The mean IQ of Americans: massive gains 1932 to 1978. *Psychol Bull* **95**, 29-51.

Frazer, Sir J. G., (1900). *The Golden Bough, a Study in Magic and Religion, Volume I: The Magic Art and the Evolution of Kings.* The MacMillan Co., London.

Gillberg, C. (1995). *Clinical Child Neuropsychiatry.* Cambridge University Press, Cambridge.

Goddard, H.H. (1912). *The Kallikak Family: A Study in the Heredity of Feeble-Mindedness.* Macmillan, New York.

Gottfredson, L.S. (1997). Why g matters: The complexity of everyday life. *Intelligence* **24**, 79-132.

Harris, J.C. (1995). *Developmental Neuropsychiatry: The Fundamentals, Volume 1.* Oxford University Press, Oxford.

Inhelder, B. (1968). *The Diagnosis of Reasoning in the Mentally Retarded.* John Day, New York.

Miller, E. (1995). Mental retardation. In: Berrios, G. and Porter, R. (Eds), *A History of Clinical Psychiatry.* Athlone Press, London, pp 212-224.

Morel, B.A. (1857). *Traité des Degénéréscences Physiques, Intellectuelles et Morales de l'Espéce Humaine et des Causes qui Produisent ces Varietés Maladie.* Baillière, Paris.

Raven, J.C. (1960). *Guide to the Standard Progressive Matrices.* H.K. Lewis, London.

Shaw, T.C. (1876). On the measurement of the palate in idiots and imbeciles. *J Ment Sci* **22**, 196-201.

Sparrow, S.S., Balla, D.A. and Cicchetti, D.V. (1984). *Interview Edition. Expanded Form Manual. Vineland Adaptive Behavior Scales.* American Guidance Service, Circle Pines, MN.

Spearman, C. (1904). "General intelligence" objectively determined and measured. *Am J Psychol* **15**, 201-293.

Sternberg, R.J. (1985). *Beyond IQ: A Triarchic Theory of Human Intelligence.* Cambridge University Press, New York.

Sternberg, R. J. (1998). *Cupid's Arrow.* Cambridge University Press, New York.

Sternberg, R.J., Castejón, J.L., Prieto, M.D., Hautamäki, J. and Grigorenko, E.L. (2001). Confirmatory factor analysis of the Sternberg Triarchic Abilities Test in three international samples: an empirical Test of the triarchic theory of intelligence. *Eur J Psychol Assessment* **17**, 1-16.

Tulsky, D.S. and Ledbetter, M.F. (2000). Updating to the WAIS-III and the WMS-III: considerations for research and clinical practice. *Psychol Assessment* **12**, 253-262.

Wechsler, D. (1974). *Manual for the Wechsler Intelligence Scale for Children-Revised*. Psychological Corporation, New York.

World Health Organisation (1992). *International Statistical Classification of Diseases and Related Health Problems, 10th revision*. World Health Organisation, Geneva.

World Health Organisation (2001a). *ICF: International Classification of Functioning, Disability and Health*. World Health Organisation, Geneva.

World Health Organisation (2001b). ICF: *Checklist Version 2.1a, Clinician Form for International Classification of Functioning, Disability and Health*. World Health Organisation, Geneva.

Learning Disability and Epilepsy: an Integrative Approach
Edited by Michael R. Trimble
© 2003 Clarius Press Ltd

2

Neuropsychiatric Epidemiology at the Interface between Learning Disability and Epilepsy

ENNAPADAM S. KRISHNAMOORTHY

*Raymond Way Neuropsychiatry Research Group, Institute of Neurology,
Queen Square, London, UK
&
TS Srinivasan Institute for Neurological Sciences and Research, Public Health
Centre, Chennai, India*

INTRODUCTION

Recent studies both community- and hospital-based have shown that there is a significant burden of psychiatric disorder in epilepsy, with as many as 50% of all subjects studied being affected. Indeed, the available epidemiological data suggests that psychiatric disorders are over-represented in epilepsy, the evidence for psychosis in particular being rather compelling (Krishnamoorthy, 2001).

The literature with regard to epilepsy and psychiatric disorder in learning-disabled populations is rather more complex. In general, there is an over-representation of both epilepsy and behaviour problems in subjects with learning disability (LD). Community studies have indicated prevalence rates of epilepsy ranging from 6% among children with mild LD (IQ 50-70) (Ross and Peckham, 1983), to 24% in severe LD (IQ <50) (Steffenberg *et al.*, 1995) and 50% in profound LD (IQ <20) (Corbett, 1988). A reasonable global estimate therefore is that between 15% (mild LD with IQ>50) and 30% (severe LD- IQ <50) of children have co-morbid epilepsy (Sillanpää, 1996).

On the other hand, it has been estimated that around 50% of subjects with LD in a hospital / institutional setting will pose management problems due to psychiatric disturbance. Affective and schizophrenic disorders, dementing syndromes, early childhood autism, hyperkinetic syndromes, neurotic, conduct and personality disorders, whether or not associated with epilepsy have been reported in this population (Reid, 1983).

ARE PSYCHIATRIC DISORDERS OVER-REPRESENTED IN SUBJECTS WITH LD AND EPILEPSY?

Given the background of high psychiatric co-morbidity in both LD and epilepsy, one would expect the burden of psychiatric co-morbidity to be significant in cases where both conditions co-exist. However, literature on psychopathology among subjects with epilepsy and LD is sparse and contradictory.

Rutter *et al.* (1970) in the Isle of Wight survey demonstrated clearly that there was an association between epilepsy and psychiatric disorder. They showed that while psychiatric morbidity was 6.6% in a control group of children, the figure rose to 11.6% with physical disorder and 34.3% with brain disorder. Further, in comparing two groups with brain lesions they also demonstrated that psychiatric co-morbidity was higher in the group with seizures (58.3%) than in the group that was seizure-free (37.5%).

Eyman *et al.* (1969) studied mentally handicapped populations in three large hospitals in the USA and reported that hyperactivity, aggression, problems with speech, and difficulties with eating / dressing were more common among institutionalised subjects with epilepsy and mental handicap. Capes and Moore (1970) compared 21 factors of maladaptive behaviour between 229 subjects with epilepsy and a non-matched control group of 511 in Arizona Children's Colony, and found significant differences in 16 out of 21 factors, hyperactivity, aggression and withdrawal in particular.

In another large population-based study, Lund (1985a) identified 324 mentally retarded adults in the county of Aarhus in Denmark, five of whom did not meet WHO criteria for mental retardation, and 17 of whom (mainly younger individuals living in the community) refused to take part. 302 individuals with mental retardation were examined with regard to epilepsy and psychiatric disorder using the Medical Research Council (MRC) schedule of handicaps, behaviours and skills (HBS) (Wing, 1980) and a schedule of psychiatric symptoms (Lund, 1985b). In 55 (18.2%) epileptic seizures had occurred some time during their lives, and in 25 (8.3%) in the last year before investigation (active epilepsy). Increasing degree of mental retardation was associated with an increased prevalence of epilepsy and psychiatric disorder. Psychiatric disorders were strongly correlated with epilepsy, with 56% of mentally handicapped persons with active epilepsy suffering from a psychiatric disorder, as compared with 26% of those without seizures, a statistically significant difference. However, this study failed to use a matched control group, which may in part explain these findings.

On the other hand Corbett (1981) in the Camberwell study did not find any significant difference in the frequency of behavioural disturbance, in comparing children with mental handicap with and without epilepsy. This latter study included patients in the community and in both hospital and non-hospital care. Deb *et al.* (1987) supported this finding when they failed to find any difference in the rates of maladaptive behaviour in a comparison of adults with epilepsy with a matched group of adults without epilepsy in a mental handicap institution. Similar findings were also reported in a study by Espie *et al.* (1989) that compared behaviour among people with mental handicap and epilepsy who lived in the community and attended day centres.

Deb and Hunter (1991 a,b,c) in a series of papers reported studies of maladaptive behaviour, psychiatric illness and personality disorders in subjects with mental handicap and epilepsy. They compared 150 subjects with mental handicap and epilepsy with a similar number of subjects with mental handicap but no epilepsy, using the Profile of Abilities and Adjustment Schedule for maladaptive behaviour. They found that while over half the total study population showed some severe maladaptive behaviour, and the problems in the epilepsy population were slightly more severe, the difference was not statistically significant.

In summary therefore, while there is little doubt that patients with LD and epilepsy have high rates of psychiatric co-morbidity (as high as 90% in some series), it is not entirely clear if an increased burden of psychiatric disorder attributable to epilepsy exists in this population.

ARE THERE SPECIFIC PATTERNS OF PSYCHIATRIC CO-MORBIDITY IN SUBJECTS WITH LD AND EPILEPSY?

Attempts to classify psychiatric disorders in children with LD and / or active epilepsy have been few. Hyperactivity, rage, antisocial behaviour and schizo-phrenia-like psychosis have all been reported, particularly in connection with temporal lobe epilepsy (Rutter *et al.*, 1970; Caplan *et al.*, 1991).

In Lund's series, the author used previously modified (for mental retarda-tion) versions of Feighner's criteria and DSM III criteria and identified an overall prevalence of 27.1%, which is lower than most other studies (Lund, 1985b). When patterns of psychopathology were compared, apart from a generic behaviour disorder category (10.9%), psychoses of uncertain type (5%), dementia and early childhood autism (3.6% each), neurosis (2%), schizophrenia (1.3%) and affective disorder (1.7%) were all identified. No cases of alcohol or drug abuse were identified in this study.

In Deb and Hunter's series (1991 a,b,c) mild to moderately impaired subjects with good communication skills who were positive on the PAA schedule for psychiatric illness were interviewed using the Present State Examination interview schedule, while those with severe mental retardation were observed and information collected from their medical notes and from the carers. Psychiatric diagnosis was made based on DSM-III-R criteria (Deb and Hunter, 1991b). Psychiatric illness was diagnosed in almost one-quarter of the population studied, but was commoner in the non-epilepsy group than in the epilepsy group, the difference being statistically significant.

There were however distinct patterns of psychiatric disorder reported in the epilepsy group, for example changeable mood, although this did not reach statistical significance. Other differences of interest were the relative absence of bipolar disorder in the epilepsy group, and the relative over-representation of non-affective psychoses in the epilepsy group, for which there is epidemiological evidence (Jalava and Sillanpää, 1996). There were also differences between community and hospital populations, behaviour such as irritability progressing to aggression being more commonly reported in the hospital population.

They also compared mild to moderately handicapped people with epilepsy and without, using the Standardised Assessment of Personality (SAP) and the T-L Personality Behaviour Inventory. They found that 26% of the entire cohort had an abnormal personality score according to the SAP schedule, and a significant proportion of these were personality disorders. The vast majority of those with high SAP scores were in-patients. However, there were no statistically significant differences between epilepsy and non-epilepsy groups (Deb and Hunter, 1991c).

In a representative population based study Steffenberg et al. (1996) identified 98 children with MR and active epilepsy, from among 48,873 children living in Gőteborg, Sweden, through multiple search procedures. The children were between 8 and 16 years of age, and of 98 identified, five had died and three declined to be examined. An experienced child neuropsychiatrist examined 90 children by interviewing the mother or principal caregiver using the Handicap, Behaviour and Skills Schedule, each interview lasting between 60 and 150 minutes. Further, each child was observed for 30 minutes. Other scales used in this study included the Childhood Autism Rating Scale and Autistic Behaviour Checklist, Asperger Syndrome Diagnostic Checklist, and Global / Social and Occupational Function Assessment Scales (GAFS & SOFAS). In addition to co-morbid psychiatric disorder, cerebral palsy, visual and hearing deficits, and self-injurious behaviour were all rated.

Fifty three (59%) out of 90 children received at least one psychiatric diagnosis. Autistic Disorder was the most common diagnosis (24/90); followed by Autistic Like Condition (10/90); Attention Deficit Hyperactivity Disorder (6/90); Asperger Syndrome, Autistic Traits and Over-anxious Disorder (3/90 each); stereotypy / habit disorder, elective mutism, conduct disorder and chronic motor tic disorder (1/90 each). Twenty eight (31%) children in this sample had self-injurious behaviour. Interestingly, a further 30 of these 90 children, many with profound mental retardation and severe communication difficulties, were classified as 'uncategorisable conditions and dementias', and only 5 of 90 subjects were declared normal. Medical syndromes (excluding epilepsy syndromes) were observed in 11 subjects, eight of whom were in the Autistic Disorder (AD) group, none in the Autistic Like Condition (ALC) group and three in the non-AD/ALC group, this difference being statistically significant (p<0.001). Psychiatric co-morbidity was generally high, with a number of patients meeting more than one diagnosis, although in some conditions such as ALC, Asperger and Autistic Traits, diagnostic criteria such as DSM were not used. This study also showed that AD in particular was associated significantly with temporal lobe epilepsy. Interestingly too, the percentages of psychiatric disorder (AD for example) were not significantly different between mild mental retardation (MMR) and severe mental retardation (SMR) groups, which is different from other series (Wing, 1993).

The authors of this study have argued elsewhere (Steffenberg and Steffenberg, 1999) that that the low prevalence of psychiatric disorder (57%) may be down to the very large proportion (almost a third) classified as 'unrecognisable condition and dementia'. Further, the finding that AD was by far the commonest psychiatric disorder, while not entirely commonplace, is supported by the strong associations between autism and epilepsy reported elsewhere (Olsson et al., 1988). The use of specific instruments targeted towards the identification of AD in this study, which has not been done in other studies, may explain this finding at least in part.

Thus, while a number of studies that have examined co-morbidity between LD and epilepsy, and LD and psychiatric disorder, in hospital, institutional and community-based populations, the literature on neuropsychiatric epidemiology at this important interface between epilepsy and LD remains rather scant.

NEUROPSYCHIATRIC EPIDEMIOLOGY AT THE INTERFACE BETWEEN EPILEPSY AND LD; WHERE DO WE GO FROM HERE?

As reviewed herein, the evidence about the relative frequency of psychiatric disorder in learning disabled populations with epilepsy is both confusing and contradictory. Further, there are a number of specific issues that have not been addressed before.

First, what we have available in the main is prevalence data from hospital, institution and a few community based studies. However, while data of this nature do inform about the public health burden of such co-morbidity, they do not help in making scientific inferences about important factors such as causality and risk. Good analytical epidemiology is required for this, and can only be achieved through well-designed and conducted cohort and case control studies, based in the population.

Second, although specific behaviour patterns have been observed, few studies have compared generic and epilepsy specific behaviours in these populations. The study of generic psychopathology is important for purposes of comparing the learning disabled population with co-morbid epilepsy, with learning disabled populations without epilepsy, and indeed non-learning disabled populations in the community. On the other hand, as demonstrated by Steffenberg *et al.* (1996), the use of instruments that can assess for specific behaviours such as the Autistic Spectrum Disorders, aggression, psychosis etc., is likely to yield rich data, and provide greater understanding about the nature and mechanisms of psychopathology at this interface. Apart from being of heuristic interest, these data have practical implications as well, with psychiatric and psychological interventions, for example, being behaviour-specific to a very great extent.

Third, it is important to note that a number of the studies have used instruments that have not been specifically developed either for epilepsy or for LD. In recent times various influential groups have been working towards building consensus in the choice of outcome measures, for example, Kerr and Espie, (1997). Appropriate measures include data-sets for aetiology and seizure type, seizure frequency, behaviour, social interaction, patient independence, contact and participation, general well being and quality of life including carer's quality of life. It has been suggested that a range of standard outcome measures be used in researching this interface, and that these should be sensitive to change, include information on individual charac-teristics, and allow for variables such as treatment compliance and environ-mental confounders. In addition there may be room for new technologies such as direct observation through computer systems and video recordings.

Fourth, there is considerable debate about the choice of psychopathology measure. In a recent review and position statement Espie *et al.* (1997) have short-listed several measures, and compared their relative attributes. The Psychopathology Instrument for Mentally Retarded Adults (Senatore *et al.*, 1985), the PASSAD [Hester Adrian Research Centre, Manchester, 1994], Aberrant Behaviour Checklist (Aman *et al.*, 1985), Psychosocial Behaviour Scale (Espie *et al.*, 1988), Adaptive Behaviour Scales- Part Two (Guess *et al.*, 1990), Attention Deficit and Hyperactivity Questionnaire (Boudreault *et al.*, 1988), Society for the Study of Behavioural Phenotypes (SSBP)- Postal Questionnaire (O'Brien, 1996) are all instruments that have been used fairly extensively in this area.

The precise choice of instrument(s) will have to be made following a careful review of the study objectives, balanced against the relative abilities and characteristics of these instruments, and pragmatic concerns. In addition to this list above, there may be some justification in including a scale for autistic behaviours following on from Steffenberg's (1996) influential paper, and a structured carer report for psychopathology such as the

Neuropsychiatric Inventory (NPI) (Cummings *et al.*, 1994). Our group for example (Krishnamoorthy *et al.*, 2000 & unpublished data) has identified specific behavioural patterns using the NPI, in an institutional population with epilepsy, and such structured carer rated information, which has not been ascertained in many previous studies, may be potentially valuable in developing interventions for LD and epilepsy.

Fifth, it has been pointed out that LD can be a state-dependent phenomenon, and thus potentially reversible (Besag, 2001). State-dependent LD can be broadly of two types - drug-induced, and epilepsy-induced. Drugs like phenobarbitone, primidone and benzodiazepines are known to cause cognitive deficits thus resulting in state-dependent LD. On the other hand, epilepsy-induced state-dependent LD may result from the ictal effects of sub-clinical seizures, focal discharges, post-ictal states, non-convulsive status, and the syndrome of Electrical Status Epilepticus in Sleep (ESES). While state-dependent LD may only form a small proportion of LD cases, its reversible nature dictates that it is examined for and carefully excluded in LD studies, including population-based studies. Screening instruments sensitive to these phenomena thus need to be developed, and incorporated into the package of diagnostic measures used.

Finally, in an ideal world, cohorts / registries of LD should be established prospectively, and include each patient who receives a diagnosis of LD. Prospective follow-up of such a cohort for co-morbid epilepsy and / or psychopathology, and nested case-control studies for risk factors, aetiology, biological and clinical correlates, quality of life, prognostic indicators, treatment response and other measures of outcome would reveal valuable epidemiologically valid information at this interface. The use of standard outcome measures as outlined previously would of course greatly aid the research process. However, this approach is tedious, expensive and long drawn out, and not surprisingly the gamut of research thus far has come from Northern Europe, where healthcare systems include the establishment and maintenance of registries.

CONCLUSIONS

In conclusion, neuropsychiatric epidemiology at the interface between LD and epilepsy is poorly researched. A better understanding about this interface would no doubt lead to focussed interventions in the community and resultant improvements in healthcare for learning – disabled populations with co-morbid epilepsy, for example Beber *et al.*, (1999). The development of consensus (Kerr and Espie, 1997); the identification of reliable and valid outcome measures and development priorities (Espie *et al.*, 1997); detailed studies based in the community (Steffenberg *et al.*, 1996); as well as recent comprehensive reviews of LD and epilepsy (Sillanpää *et al.*, 1999), have set the stage for high quality research efforts at this interface, which we hope will follow in the years that come.

REFERENCES

Aman, M.N., Singh, N.N., Stewart, A.W. and Field, C.J. (1985). The Aberrant Behaviour Checklist: a behaviour rating scale for the assessment of treatment effects. *Am J Ment Def* **89**, 485-491.

Beber, E., Bailey, N.M. and Cooper, S.A. (1999). Health gain for epilepsy associated with learning disabilities psychiatric care. *Ir J Psych Med* **16**(2), 46-50.

Besag, F.M.C. (2001). Treatment of state-dependent learning disability. *Epilepsia* **42** (Suppl 1), 52-54.

Boudreault, M., Thivierge, J., Coter, R., Boutin, P., Julien, Y. and Bergeron, S. (1988). Cognitive development and reading achievement in pervasive-ADD, situational-ADD, and control children. *J Child Psychol Psychiatry* **29**, 611-619.

Capes, L. and Moore, B.C. (1970). Behaviour differences between seizure and non-seizure retardates. *Arizona Med* **27**, 74-76.

Caplan, R., Shields, W.R., Mori, L. and Yudovin, S. (1991). Middle childhood onset of interictal psychosis. *J Am Acad Child Adolesc Psychiatry* **30**, 893-896.

Corbett, J.A. (1988). Epilepsy and mental handicap. In: Laidlaw, J., Richens, A. and Oxley, J. (Eds), *A Textbook of Epilepsy*. Churchill Livingstone, Edinburgh, pp. 533-538.

Corbett, J.A., (1981). Epilepsy and mental retardation. In: Trimble, M.R. and Reynolds, E.H. (Eds), *Epilepsy and Psychiatry*. Churchill Livingstone, Edinburgh, pp. 138-146.

Cummings, J.L., Mega, M., Gray, K., Rosenberg-Thompson, S., Carusi, D.A. and Gornbein, J. (1994). The Neuropsychiatric Inventory: comprehensive assessment of psychopathology in dementia. *Neurology* **44**, 2308-2314.

Deb, S., Cowie, V.A. and Richens, A. (1987). Folate metabolism and problem behaviour in mentally handicapped epileptics. *J Ment Def Res* **31**, 163-168.

Deb, S. and Hunter, D. (1991a). Psychopathology of People with Mental Handicap and Epilepsy. I: Maladaptive Behaviour. *Br J Psychiatry* **159**, 822-826.

Deb, S. and Hunter, D. (1991b). Psychopathology of People with Mental Handicap and Epilepsy. II: Psychiatric Illness. *Br J Psychiatry* **159**, 826-830.

Deb, S. and Hunter, D. (1991c). Psychopathology of People with Mental Handicap and Epilepsy. III: Personality Disorder. *Br J Psychiatry* **159**, 830-834.

Espie, C.A., Pashley, E.S., Bonham, K.G., Sourindham, I. and O'Donovan, M. (1989). The mentally handicapped person with epilepsy: a comparative study investigating psychosocial functioning. *J Ment Def Res* **33**, 123-135.

Espie, C.A., Kerr, M., Paul, A., O'Brien, G. *et al.* (1997). Learning disability and epilepsy. 2. A review of available outcome measures and position statement on development priorities. *Seizure* **6**, 337-350.

Espie, C.A., Montgomery, J.A. and Gillies, J.B. (1988). The development of a psychosocial behaviour scale for the assessment of mentally handicapped people. *J Ment Def Res* **32**, 395-403.

Eyman, R.K., Capes, L., Moore, B.C. *et al.* (1969). Retardates with seizures. *Am J Ment Def* **74**, 651-659.

Guess, D., Siegel-Causey, E., Roberts, S., Rues, J., Thompson, B. and Siegel-Causey, D. (1990). Assessment and analysis of behavioural state and related variables among students with profoundly handicapping conditions. *Journal of the Association for Persons with Severe Handicaps* **15**, 211-230.

Jalava, M. and Sillanpää, M. (1996). Concurrent illnesses in adults with childhood-onset epilepsy: a population-based 35-year follow-up study. *Epilepsia* **37** (12), 1155-1163.

Kerr, M.P. and Espie, C.A. (1997). Learning disability and epilepsy: 1. Towards common outcome measures. *Seizure* **6**, 331-336.

Krishnamoorthy, E.S. (2001). Psychiatric issues in epilepsy. *Curr Opin Neurol*, **14**(2), 217-224.

Krishnamoorthy, E.S., Brown, R.J., Samuel, R. and Trimble, M.R. (2000). The Neuropsychiatric Inventory in Epilepsy. *Epilepsia*, **41** (Suppl Florence), 155.

Lund, J. (1985a). Epilepsy and psychiatric disorder in the mentally retarded adult. *Acta Psychiatr Scand* **71**, 557-562.

Lund, J. (1985b). The prevalence of psychiatric morbidity in mentally retarded adults. *Acta Psychiatr Scand* **72**, 563-570.

O'Brien, G. (1996). A comparative study of young children and adults with Fragile X Syndrome. *Genetic Counselling* **7**, 167.

Olsson, I., Steffenberg, S. and Gillberg, C. (1988). Epilepsy and autism and autistic-like conditions: a population-based study. *Arch Neurol* **45**, 666-668.

Reid, A.H. (1983). Psychiatry of mental handicap: a review. *J Roy Soc Med* **76**, 587-592.

Ross, E.M. and Peckham, C.S. (1983). School children with epilepsy. In: Parsonage, M., Grant, R.H.E. and Craig, A.G. (Eds), *Advances in Epileptology; XIV Epilepsy International Symposium*. Raven Press, New York, pp. 213-220.

Rutter, M., Graham, P. and Yule, W. (1970). *A Neuropsychiatric Study in Childhood*. Heinemann Medical, London.

Senatore, V., Matson, J.L. and Kazdin, A.E. (1985). An inventory to assess psychopathology of mentally retarded adults. *Am J Ment Defic* **89**(5), 459-466.

Sillanpää, M. (1996). Epilepsy in the mentally retarded. In: Wallace, S. (Ed), *Epilepsy in Children*. Chapman and Hall, London, pp. 417-427.

Sillanpää, M., Gram, L., Johannessen, S.I. and Tomson, T. (1999). (Eds), *Epilepsy and Mental Retardation*. Wrightson Biomedical, Petersfield.

Steffenberg, E. and Steffenberg, S. (1999). Epilepsy and other neuropsychiatric morbidity in mentally retarded children. In: Sillanpää, M., Gram, L., Johannessen, S., I. and Tomson, T. (Eds), *Epilepsy and Mental Retardation*. Wrightson Biomedical, Petersfield, pp. 47-59.

Steffenberg, S., Gillberg, C. and Steffenberg, U. (1996). Psychiatric disorders in children and adolescents with mental retardation and active epilepsy. *Arch Neurol* **53**, 904-912.

Steffenberg, U., Hagberg, G. and Kyllerman, M. (1995). Active epilepsy in mentally retarded children. *Acta Paediatr Scand* **84**, 1153-1159.

Wing, L. (1980). The MRC handicaps, behaviour and skills (HBS) schedule. In: Stromgren, E., Dupont, A. and Nielsen, J.A. (Eds), *Epidemiological Research as Basis for Organisation in Extramural Psychiatry. Acta Psychiatr Scand* **62**, 241-247.

Wing, L. (1993). The definition and prevalence of autism: a review. *Eur Child Adolesc Psychiatry* **2**, 61-74.

Learning Disability and Epilepsy: an Integrative Approach
Edited by Michael R. Trimble
© 2003 Clarius Press Ltd

3

The Genetics of Learning Disorders

MATTI SILLANPÄÄ[*] AND JAANA LÄHDETIE[**]

[*]Departments of Child Neurology and Public Health, Turku University,
Turku, Finland
[**]Department of Medical Genetics, Turku University, Turku,
and Rinnekoti Foundation, Espoo, Finland

INTRODUCTION

The medical identification of learning disorder (LD) must always be followed by aetiological assessment. Several classifications of the causes of LD have been developed based, for example, on presumed timing of the insult, mechanism of action of the cause, autopsy studies, and neuroradiological studies. LD results from an unsuccessful interplay between genes and environment in the development of the human brain and its cognitive skills. Even in case of a single known genetic aetiological factor, such as trisomy 21, the phenotypic effects and level of LD may be variable due to multifactorial and environmental influences. On the other hand, in patients with a non-genetic factor such as alcohol exposure in utero, genetic susceptibility may modify the clinical symptoms and severity of LD. On an individual level, despite the advances of genetic methods, it is often difficult to find how much the cause of LD is inherited and how much acquired.

The detection of the chromosomal abnormality in Down's syndrome (Lejeune et al., 1959) led to the wide use of cytogenetic methodology and opened doors to novel techniques to explore the genetic background of LD. Based on the rapid development of genetic, and neuro-imaging methods, the aetiology can now be clarified in the vast majority of patients with severe LD (Fryers, 1984; Steffenberg et al., 1995; Arvio and Sillanpää, 2003).

In patients with mild LD, the spectrum of aetiologies is different from that of severe LD, with more frequent untraceable and less frequent acquired aetiologies (Steffenberg et al., 1995; Stromme, 2000). There is a hypothesis that multiple additive genes are responsible for mild LD, but it has been questioned (Åkesson, 1986).

In recent population-based studies, genetic aetiologies cover 28-38% of all causes of LD (Matilainen *et al.*, 1995; Hou *et al.*, 1998; Stromme *et al.*, 2002). The known genetic aetiologies can be divided into three groups: (1) chromosomal abnormalities, (2) single gene disorders, and (3) miscellaneous disorders. This grouping, however, meets some problems because, for example, microdeletions are grouped into chromosomal abnormalities, though the smallest deletions overlap with single gene disorders. The miscellaneous group consists of known clinical syndromes with suspected but yet unknown genetic aetiology, complex traits (i.e. polygenic or multifactorial inheritance) and non-syndromic (often familial) LDs with suspected but unknown inheritance. Owing to the rapid progress in the human genome project, more and more specific genetic aetiologies for many LDs are being discovered and multiple loci responsible for polygenic traits are being unravelled.

GENETIC METHODS AS DIAGNOSTIC TOOLS

The genetic aetiology of LD should be assessed by starting with a good medical history. This includes the construction of a family tree in three successive generations, and questions on spontaneous abortions, stillbirths, neonatal deaths, malformations, and possible consanguinity of the parents of a proband. The subsequent medical examination consists of a thorough clinical evaluation with special emphasis on dysmorphic features, skin pigmentation irregularities, congenital abnormalities of the heart, kidneys and other organs, growth curves, and hearing and vision. A good neurological clinical examination is also needed. Photographs or videofilms of the patient may prove invaluable for identification of specific syndromes. A clinical geneticist may suggest syndromes when seeing the patient and by the help of dysmorphology database searches. Radiological examinations such as ultrasound or X-ray may be needed in some cases to confirm a suspected anomaly. At least one high-resolution brain MRI examination is also necessary to be able to detect structural brain abnormalities.

Cytogenetics

Chromosome analysis is a basic tool in the evaluation of a patient with LD. Even in patients whose clinical diagnosis is evident, such as in Down's syndrome, the karyotype must be analysed in order to distinguish ordinary trisomies from those with a translocation of chromosome 21 to another chromosome. The human genome consists of 23 pairs of chromosomes, that can be visualised in a light microscope in metaphase spreads. Peripheral blood lymphocytes are cultured in the presence of mitogen, arrested at metaphase, spread on slides and stained with specific stains. The most common staining used is G-banding which yields about 350-400 bands per haploid genome (23 chromosomes).

The standard karyotype is a result of the analysis of at least 20 metaphases per patient. The level of resolution is often sufficient for detection of major chromosomal abnormalities such as numerical aberrations (e.g. trisomies), large deletions or duplications, marker chromosomes and mosaicisms.

The high resolution karyotype is needed when the standard karyotype is normal and there is strong suspicion of a chromosomal disorder based on the clinical findings or on pedigree data. This gives a resolution at 550-850 bands per haploid genome which allows detection of small deletions, duplications or inversions. High-resolution banding is a very laborious method and should be restricted to selected patients, if possible, after consulting a clinical geneticist.

If there is a suspicion of mosaicism, the chromosome analysis can be performed on tissue other than lymphocytes, e.g. fibroblasts from a skin biopsy. Sometimes a small unbalanced translocation may be indirectly detected if the chromosomes of a healthy parent are found to carry a balanced translocation which may be more easily visualised. If a prenatal karyotype has been done using chorionic villi, amniocentesis or cord blood, the result is reliable for trisomies and other large chromosomal abnormalities, but repeated karyotyping from peripheral blood is recommended on a child who shows clear dysmorphic features in addition to LD.

FISH karyotyping methods.

Introduction of a set of probes for all the sub-telomeric sequences for all the different human chromosomes on a single test slide allowed the simultaneous fluorescent in situ hybridisation (FISH) analysis of these abnormalities. Spectral karyotyping (SKY) refers to another fluorescence in situ hybridisation - based novel technique taking advantage of chromosome-specific painting probes. These methods seem to become necessary tools for investigation of the genetic aetiology of LD, especially when dysmorphic features are present (Clarkson *et al.*, 2002).

Since the clinical features related to the various small deletions and duplications are very variable, these methods serve as a good screen for such syndromes. One problem limiting the use of these tests is the relatively high cost.

Microdeletions are detectable using specific DNA probes that hybridise to the locus of interest in the chromosomes on a metaphase spread. Using fluorescent labels the presence (normal result) or absence (microdeletion) of a signal in one of the two homologous chromosomes can be observed with a fluorescence microscope. A reference probe is used to verify the quality of hybridisation. The method is useful for such syndromes as CATCH-22, Williams syndrome and Smith-Magenis syndrome, whereas in Prader-Willi and Angelman syndromes, of which part of the mutations are uniparental disomies, not deletions, the DNA tests are recommended.

Molecular methods

DNA analysis

A specific DNA test, if available, gives the confirmation of the suspected monogenic disease if a mutation can be detected. Mutation detection may proceed in different ways that depend on the size of the gene, the number and incidence of known mutations and the usefulness of the test method. Most methods use genomic DNA extracted from peripheral blood, although other sources of DNA such as buccal smears and blood smears (Guthrie cards) may also be used. Amplification of the genomic sequences studied using the polymerase chain reaction (PCR) is normally the starting point of the molecular analysis.

The second phase of a DNA test has various technical alternatives and novel innovations are done continuously in this field. Restriction enzymes may be used to analyze the size of the amplified gene by Southern hybridization e.g. in detection of an amplification of a repeated sequence. Since restriction enzymes cut the DNA strand at specific DNA sequences, they can also be used for detection of point mutations in cases where the specific mutation is known (e.g. based on analysis of other patients in the same family or population). Deletions may be screened by a multiplex PCR method: several exonic sequences are amplified simultaneously and lack of amplification show the deletion. In Duchenne muscular dystrophy (DMD) which often includes LD the test detects approximately 70% of all mutations.

Since many monogenic diseases show a large number of different mutations of the same gene, it may be necessary to sequence the whole gene (normally the exons of the gene). For very large genes such as the NF1 gene, however, sequencing is often considered too laborious whereas for smaller genes such as the ARX-gene the mutations of which cause X-linked mental retardation (Bienvenu et al., 2002), sequencing of the whole gene is easier. Semi-automated DNA sequencers have become part of the armament of clinical laboratories in addition to research laboratories. To facilitate the recognition and isolation of a mutated versus normal allele, denaturing gel electrophoresis may be used prior to sequencing.

The molecular test to detect the fragile X syndrome is based on analysis of the size of the (CGG) trinucleotide repeat flanking the FMR1 gene. The normal stable repeat varies between 5 to 60 repeats, and the most common alleles in normal people are 29 and 30 repeats. A premutation is an expansion of 60-230 repeats size and does not cause LD. The gene function is normal and carriers are healthy. The premutation is labile and when inherited from the mother, tends to expand further in the maternal meiosis, especially if the premutation is larger than 90 repeats. The full mutation is an expansion of at least 230 repeats, sometimes more than 1000 repeats. It causes methylation of a CpG island flanking the gene and subsequently inactivation of the gene.

In boys this causes the fragile-X syndrome and approximately half of the girls with a full mutation are affected by LD.

Polymorphic DNA markers such as di-, tri-, or tetranucleotide repeats, or single nucleotide polymorphisms (SNP) can be used to screen the whole genome for deletions, duplications, uniparental disomies or other rearrangements that escape cytogenetic detection (this may be called fluorescent genotyping). Also a set of telomeric DNA markers can be used to detect subtelomeric alterations as an alternative to cytogenetic FISH methods. The markers can be selected to screen the X-chromosome if LD shows X-linked inheritance but is not caused by the FMR1 gene. Linkage studies may be helpful for genetic counselling purposes but require DNA samples from a large number of family members. Linkage studies combined with positional cloning methods allow researchers to isolate the gene and to identify mutations responsible for LD, as e.g. in primary microcephaly (Bond et al., 2002).

DNA microarrays (chips) are future diagnostic tools which allow simultaneous analysis of numerous DNA sequences with probes fixed on a solid support, e.g. a microscope slide.

RNA and protein analysis

The identification of a mutation at the DNA level may be technically too laborious for clinical purposes and therefore, alternative methods based on the analysis of the gene products, i.e. the mRNA and the protein may applied. RNA may be extracted from peripheral blood lymphocytes or an established lymphoblastoid cell line. The expression of the gene is analysed by reverse transcriptase PCR (RT-PCR) and Northern blotting. A problem is that the expression of the gene may be limited to brain tissue and cannot be studied in lymphocyte preparations. Microarrays for gene expression studies are a novel, evolving technology where the clinical applications are promising but still rare.

Protein expression can be studied by antibodies using e.g. Western blotting, ELISA or other immunological techniques. Lack of the dystrophin protein in a muscle biopsy of a DMD patient can be observed using immunostaining. In Fragile X syndrome the expression of the FMR protein is prevented by the mutation of the FMR1 gene. The FMR1 antibody test was found to be suitable for screening among a large population of retarded males using blood smears (deVries et al., 1998). Microarray immunoassay methods are also evolving.

Enzymatic and other biochemical studies

The mutation may not cause the loss of a gene product but may impair the function of the protein. This may be seen as a reduction or lack of the enzyme activity. In many mitochondrial encephalopathies the gene defect may be difficult to discern due to the multitude of subunits of proteins and nuclear genes coding for them. Instead, it may be possible to show a defect in one of the complexes of the respiratory chain using fresh *muscle biopsy* material.

Different types of *blood tests* are useful for diagnosis of specific syndromes. Lysosomal storage material can be observed as vacuoles in lymphocytes in blood smears. In addition to changes in electrolyte and acid-base balance, the levels of lactate and pyruvate often are abnormal in many disorders of energy metabolism, copper and coeruloplasmin are low in Wilson's disease, blood desialotransferrin levels are high in carbohydrate deficient glycoprotein syndrome, blood phytanic acid and very long chain fatty acid levels are increased in adrenoleukodystrophy, etc.

Urinary analyses are used as screens for many metabolic diseases.

Glycoproteoglycans, oligosaccharides, aminoacids and organic acids can be analysed.

Specific *analyses of cerebrospinal fluid* such as analysis of lactate or amino acids may sometimes be needed for diagnostic purposes.

CHROMOSOMAL ABNORMALITY SYNDROMES

In live births, approx. 0.4-0.5% have a major chromosomal anomaly associated with LD. Chromosomal abnormalities comprise 33-43% of all genetic causes of LD (Hou et al., 1998). Any abnormal events in the first, second or third trimester, small for gestational age birth weight and post-maturity increase the risk for a chromosomal abnormality. Typical features in chromosomal anomalies associated with LD include dysmorphism, congenital abnormalities in multiple organ systems, intrauterine or postnatal growth retardation, and endocrine disturbances.

Trisomies

The incidence of *trisomy 21* (Down's syndrome), probably known since 1846 and first distinctly described as a nosological entity in 1866 by Down, is approx. 1 in 600 births (Down, 1866). As in most trisomies, the increasing incidence is associated with increasing maternal age. More than 90% present with an extra chromosome 21, and 8% are associated with a translocation chromosome 21 to another chromosome. About one fifth of the patients are less than 2500g by birthweight. They have a small brachycephalic skull, typical dysmorphic facial appearance with upslanting palpebral fissures with a complete medial epicanthal fold, Brushfield spots, low nose ridge, hypoplasia of facial bones, micrognathia, and low-set, small and mis-shapen ears. Congenital malformations, especially heart anomalies (ventricular or atrial septal defect, Fallot's tetralogy) occur in 40%. Abnormalities in gastrointestinal system (oesophago-tracheal atresia, duodenal stenosis, Hirschsprung's disease) are the second most common group of malformations (in 20%). Other typical features include osseous (decrease of acetabular and iliac angles, narrowing of the cervical canal, atlantoaxial subluxation) (in 10-20%), cutaneous (e.g. hyperkeratotic lesions, alopecia areata and alteration of vasomotor control), and haematopoietic and/or immunological abnormalities. The latter include an increased risk for leukaemia, lymphatic malignancies and infections and autoimmune diseases such as hypothyroidism, diabetes mellitus, rheumatoid arthritis and coeliac disease.

LD is a striking characteristic of Down's syndrome. The intelligence level ranges from mild to moderate, with better visual and social processing than auditory processing. Muscular hypotonia is marked and may cause feeding difficulties in infancy. Although the incidence of epilepsy is lower than in many other LD syndromes, infantile spasms are more common than expected in Down's syndrome (Pollack *et al.*, 1978). Aging is often accompanied by Alzheimer-like dementia and associated epilepsy.

Trisomy 13 (Patau syndrome) occurs in 1 in 10,000 births. LD is severe. The syndrome presents with microphthalmia, bilateral cleft lip and palate or other types of facial clefts, hexadactyly and other supernumerary fingers and toes. Heart disease is present in 80% and kidney disease in 30-50%. Accordingly, the diagnosis of trisomy 13 is obvious, when severe LD is associated with holoprocencephaly and visceral and limb malformations.

Trisomy 18 (Edwards syndrome). The incidence is 1 in 5,000 births. A marked intrauterine growth retardation is associated with heart and various cerebral anomalies. Distal abnormalities include finger contractions, closed fists, 'trigger thumb', and hallux malleus with 'rocker bottom feet'. Fifty per cent have gross cerebral anomalies resulting from a defective rhombencephalic development, and 80% have widespread heterotopias. LD is severe.

Trisomy mosaicism

Complete trisomies 8 and 9 are only possible in neonates as mosaics. Trisomy 8 (Warkany syndrome) has the incidence of approx. 1 in 25,000. The birthweight is usually normal. Craniofacial dysmorphism with a typical thick lower lip, osteoarticular deformities, visceral changes and dermatoglyphic characteristics are typical of this syndrome. Absent or dysplastic patellae may be present. Agenesis of the corpus callosum is the most remarkable anomaly. LD is moderate to severe. Trisomy mosaicism may also be associated with trisomies 13, 18 and 21. Less than 5% of patients with trisomy 21 are mosaics. There appearance is less abnormal than in normal Down's syndrome. In non-symptomatic adults who have Down offspring, a mild trisomy mosaicism can be detected.

Deletion and duplication disorders

The group is very heterogenous. In about one third, there is a balanced translocation or inversion in a carrier parent but, in the vast majority, the cases are mutations. Almost any chromosome may be affected and their telomeres are particularly involved in microdeletions and macrodeletions.

1p36 deletion syndrome is probably the most common telomeric deletion, with the incidence of 1 in 5,000. The syndrome is characterized by deep-set eyes, narrow palpebral fissures, and mid-face dysplasia, epilepsy and severe LD.

Wolf-Hirschhorn syndrome occurs in about 1 in 25,000 births and is characterized by microcephaly, dysmorphic nasal ridge, arched eyebrows, hypertelorism and prominent glabella ('Greek warrior helmet sign'). LD is commonly associated with epilepsy. LD is severe and associated with indifference to pain and also to social stimuli. The syndrome is caused by a deletion of the short arm of chromosome 4, often the band p16.3 only.

Cri du chat syndrome. The incidence is 1 in 20,000 births. Characteristic of the syndrome is a weak mewing cry, round, faunlike face, microcephalia, micrognathia, and broadened nasal ridge. The life expectancy is shortened by LD, heart disease, upper motor neuron disease and epileptic seizures. LD is usually severe. The cause is a deletion of the short arm of chromosome 5.

18q deletion syndrome. The incidence is approx. 1 in 40,000 live births. The syndrome is one of the most common segmental aneusomies compatible with life. It presents with failure to thrive, short stature, muscular hypotonia, hearing loss associated with a stenosed external auditory canal and dysmyelination of white matter tracts in brain imaging studies.

CATCH 22 syndrome occurs in 1 in 5,000 births. It includes three clinically defined syndromes: the diGeorge, velocardiofacial and conotruncal anomaly face syndromes. The acronym CATCH22 derives from the phrase CATCH 22, which was used by Joseph Heller as the title of his book but also stands for Cardiac defects, Abnormal facial features, T cell deficit due to thymic hypoplasia, Cleft palate, and Hypocalcemia due to hypoparathyroidism. LD is mostly mild. The abnormality is deletion of the band q11.22 in the chromosome 22 and the phenotypic variability is associated with the size and location of the deletion.

Miller-Dieker syndrome is identified by neuroimaging studies in patients with microcephalia and severe LD as a Type I lissencephaly with few or no cortical gyri and diffusely thickened cerebral cortex. LD is severe. A microdeletion is in the band p13.3 of the chromosome 17.

Smith-Magenis syndrome. The features of the syndrome are hearing impairment, involuntary movements, hoarse voice, marked nocturnal restlessness, and LD. The microdeletion is situated in the band p11.2 of the chromosome 17.

Williams syndrome. Few estimates exist on the incidence of this disorder. One estimate is 1 in 7,500 live births (Stromme *et al.*, 2002). The syndrome is displayed by an elfin face, short stature, typical dental malformations, cardiovascular abnormalities (mostly supravalvular or other stenosis) (Eronen *et al.*, 2002), hoarse voice, marked visuospatial cognitive problems, and a typical personality that includes overfriendliness, anxiety and attention deficit. LD is moderate or severe. The syndrome is caused by a microdeletion in the band q11.23 of the chromosome 7. The diagnosis is made using the FISH method based on the demonstration of the disappearance of elastin gene.

Uniparental disomies

The exceptional inheritance of two homologous chromosomes from only one parent is called uniparental disomy. Dependent on parental or maternal monoallelically active genes, i.e. genomic imprinting, the disomy may lead to an imbalanced expression of these imprinted genes and cause a clinically relevant abnormality. A typical example is the contrast between Prader-Willi and Angelman syndromes.

Prader-Willi syndrome occurs in 1 in 10,000-25,000 births (Lee, 2002). The syndrome is highly suggestive in the newborn who is born by breech delivery at term, is small for gestational age, shows profound muscular hypotonia, and has swallowing difficulties necessitating tube feeding. During the first years of life, the feeding problems and slender body shape turn to hyperphagia and obesity. Their later age is characterised by persistent hypotonia, short stature, acromicria, cryptorchidism, genital hypoplasia, and diabetes mellitus and cardiovascular complications secondarily to obesity. Behavioural features include unexpected temper tantrums and picking of their skin and other types of self-injurious behaviour. Most patients have mild to moderate LD. The most common genetic abnormality is deletion of the bands q11.2-q13 of the paternal chromosome 15, but some originate from the maternal uniparental disomy.

Angelman syndrome (a previous epithet was 'happy puppet syndrome') is estimated to occur in 1 in 20,000 births (Galvan Manso *et al.*, 2002). Contrary to Prader-Willi syndrome, the identification of Angelman syndrome in the neonatal period may be difficult. Slow gross motor development, ataxia, cheerful mood with inappropriate bursts of laughter, restlessness and hyperactivity, epileptic seizures, absence of language, and marked LD with autistic features are suggestive. Microcephaly, wildly spaced teeth, blond hairs, prognathism, coarse facial features, joint contractures and scoliosis may occur. Approximately 95% have the same chromosomal abnormality as in Prader-Willi syndrome but inherited from the maternal side. Both the location of abnormality and uniparental disomy can be ascertained with DNA analysis.

Other uniparental disomies. Many rare syndromes with a uniparental disomy have been reported. Newborns with Beckwith-Wiedemann syndrome have high birth weight and later high height and weight, macroglossia and an umbilical hernia. LD is mostly mild or moderate. The abnormality is located in the short arm of the paternal chromosome 11. In some patients, the Silver-Russell syndrome, with short stature and LD, is associated with the disomy of maternal chromosome 7.

Balanced translocations and inversions

Translocations are cytogenetically divided into two groups: centred or Robertsonian translocations of two chromosomes with an acrocentric location of centromere (chromosomes 13, 14, 15, 21 and 22) and reciprocal translocations with breakage of chromatids and an error-free or erroneous repair of the two broken chromosome ends. The translocation is called balanced when the ligation of the two chromatids takes place without loss or insertion of chromosomal material whereas it is called unbalanced in cases where a fragment of the chromosome is lost or gained during the repair process. The resolution is, however, at the cytogenetic level and it is known that small fragments of DNA may be lost during the formation of a chromosomal rearrangement. Inversion refers to breakage of a chromosome at two distinct sites and inversion of the fragment in between the sites without loss of chromosomal material. Carriers of balanced translocations and inversions are usually completely healthy, but they may have some problems with fertility and they have an increased risk of having offspring with unbalanced karyotypes. Analysis of a larger number of patients with different balanced translocations and LD has proven a good starting point in mapping genes for LD.

In a balanced carrier of the Robertsonian translocation, the number of chromosomes decreases to 45. The most common Robertson translocation is t(13;14). The incidence of carriers is 1 in 1,500. Theoretically, these carriers have a great risk for trisomy 13 offspring, but virtually only 5% of pregnancies present with this trisomy. A rarer centric translocation t(14;21) bears a risk of trisomy 21 in 5% of offspring when the father is carrier and 20% when the mother is carrier. An unbalanced form is found in approximately 5% of patients with Down's syndrome.

Unbalanced reciprocal translocations cause lethality or various developmental disorders. If very large fragments are translocated, the carrier of the balanced form may suffer from reduced fertility or miscarriage in early pregnancy. When the translocation is between small chromosomal fragments, the risk for severe LD together with other congenital anomalies is generally larger, although there are differences between different translocations. Inversions cause errors during meiosis and may lead to deletions, i.e. developmental disorders in the offspring.

Sex chromosome disorders

Sex chromosome disorders are associated with LD only in cases of tetrasomy or pentasomy. Boys who have Klinefelter syndrome with karyotype 48,XXXY or 49,XXXXY almost invariably have LD and urogenital or other malformations. A karyotype of 48,XXYY has a similar phenotype with hypogonadism, delayed puberty, tall height and LD. All these syndromes are very rare.

MONOGENIC DISEASES

The number of identified single gene LD diseases with mendelian inheritance is steadily increasing, but many of them are very rare. The number of different LD syndromes with autosomal inheritance can be estimated to be 2,000-3,000. Dominantly inherited LD syndromes include e.g. neurofibromatosis, tuberous sclerosis and the Sotos syndrome. The number of autosomal recessive diseases is high and the genes encode for proteins involved in the growth and function of neurons, and most are rare neurometabolic diseases. The number of known X-chromosomal recessive loci causing LD in boys is increasing (Bardoni and Mandel, 2002; Bienvenu *et al.*, 2002). Of them, the most common is Fragile-X syndrome. X-chromosomal dominant genes may be responsible for some forms of LD syndromes in girls, such as incontinentia pigmenti and Rett's syndrome.

Autosomal dominant LD diseases

Neurofibromatosis type I (von Recklinghausen disease, peripheral neurofibromatosis) is the most common autosomal dominant monogenic disease. The incidence is variable, usually 1 in 3,500 births. Six or more café-au-lait spots of 0.5 to several centimetres, two or more neurofibromas, axillary freckling, one plexiform neuroma, two or more iris hamartomas (Lisch nodules), optic glioma, typical osseous lesions such as sphenoid dysplasia or tibial pseudoarthrosis, and one or more first degree relative are typical features. Two or more of these criteria must be present to justify the diagnosis of neurofibromatosis type 1. Café-au-lait spots, plexiform neurofibroma, and pseudoarthrosis are usually first to occur, followed by axillary freckling, Lisch nodules and neurofibromas. About half the patients have mild LD, but the intelligence level is in most cases normal. The gene defect maps to the chromosome 17q11.2. Mutations are common and expressivity of the gene is greatly variable even in the same pedigree. Life average expectancy is shortened to 61 years, mainly due to malignancy and cardiovascular complications (Zoller *et al.*, 1995).

Another type, *neurofibromatosis type II* or central neurofibromatosis has the incidence of 1 in 87,000 births and is featured by bilateral acoustic neurinomas (schwannomas) in about 90%, meningeomas in 50% and, rarely, ependymomas and gliomas. The inheritance is autosomal dominant, and the gene defect is located in the chromosome 22q11.2. The mutation frequency is high.

Tuberous sclerosis. The incidence estimate is 1 in 5,800 live births. Typical features include cutaneous manifestations such as facial angiofibromas (in 85%), hypopigmentation spots (80%), periungual fibromas (50%), shagreen patches (40-50%), and fibrous plaques of forehead (25%). Hypopigmentation spots may in early infancy only be seen with a Wood light but soon come visible in day light. Visceral abnormalities include renal, cardiac and ophthalmologic tumours, usually hamartomas, rhabdomyomas or lipomas. Cerebral tuberi can be detected in 80-90% in neuroimaging studies. In 50-70%, dental enamel abnormalities can be found. Epileptic seizures including infantile spasms occur in 80-90% and LD in 50%. Two gene defects have been identified, one in chromosome 9q34 producing hamartin, and another in chromosome 16p13 producing tuberin. Gene mutations vary markedly (in approx. 70%) from pedigree to pedigree on both paternally and maternally derived tuberous sclerosis alleles, in contract to many other genetic diseases. This must be considered in genetic counselling (Roberts *et al.*, 2002).

Rubinstein-Taybi syndrome. The incidence in the general population is not known but the prevalence in LD clinics is about 1 in 600. The syndrome can be identified in the neonatal period from broad thumbs and halluces, and the facial abnormalities. In the meta-analysis of 732 cases, 18 different chromosomal anomalies were found (Cantani and Gagliesi, 1998). The gene locus is assigned to chromosome 16p.13.3. Microdeletions, translocations, and inversions can be found in that locus. Disruption of the human CREB (cyclic AMP-responsive element binding protein), a nuclear protein participating as a coactivator in cyclic AMP-regulated gene expression, leads to the Rubinstein-Taybi syndrome by either gross chromosomal rearrangements (20% microdeletions or truncating mutations) or by point mutations (Taine *et al.*, 1998).

Sotos syndrome. This syndrome is characterized by excessively rapid physical growth, advanced bone age, acromegalic features, and a nonprogressive cerebral disorder with LD. The gene mutation is in NSD1 on chromosome 5q35 (Kurotaki *et al.*, 2002). The majority of the cases are sporadic.

Autosomal recessive LD diseases

Neurometabolic storage diseases frequently cause a progressive LD. Their percentage of all the LD population is, however, small. Among 306 adults, resident in an institution for the mentally retarded and screened for LD, the cause was considered as a metabolic disorder in only 1.6% (Van Buggenhout *et al.*, 2001).

Phenylketonuria. Lysosomal diseases include more than 60 entities, but only a part of them lead to LD. One of the most common is phenylketonuria. Its incidence varies from 1 in 4,000 in Ireland to 1 in 100,000 in Japan and among African Americans. In Finland, there are only 10 ascertained cases during the last 40 years. Storage of phenylalanine into the brain results from a lack of phenylalanine hydroxylase and subsequent defective hydroxylation of phenylalanine to tyrosine. In the gene encoding phenylalanine hydroxylase, mutations are common (Mirisola *et al.*, 2001), and their presence is reflected in various degrees of hyperalaninaemia.

Aspartylgucosaminuria is an autosomal recessive lysosomal disease caused by a deficiency of the enzyme aspartylglucosaminidase. A specific mutation is concentrated in Finland, and the incidence of the disease has been estimated to be 1 in 18,000. Recurrent infections, and inguinal and umbilical hernias in infancy are followed by delayed psychomotor development, behavioural abnormalities, coarse facial features and hoarse voice. The diagnosis is mostly made at preschool age based on very high aspartylglucosamine concentration in urine. The gene error, the AGU-Fin major mutation, is located in the long arm of chromosome 4 and is responsible for 98% of Finnish cases. The estimates for carrier frequency vary between 1:30 and 1:80.

Neuronal ceroid lipofuscinoses constitute the vast majority of progressive central nervous system diseases in childhood worldwide. They have one feature in common, viz. storage of autofluorescent waxy pigments in neurons and other tissues. Neuronal ceroid lipofuscinoses are caused by various gene defects.

The infantile form is particularly common in Finland with the incidence of 1 in 20,000. The onset of symptoms is at the age of 7 to 20 months leading rapidly to motor and mental deterioration, severe visual defect, epilepsy and spasticity. The disease is caused by a mutation in the gene located in the chromosome 1p32 and encoding the enzyme palmityl protein esterase 1. Mutations of the same gene have been found in some patients with a late-infantile, juvenile and even adult ceroid lipofuscinosis.

Late-infantile neuronal ceroid lipofuscinosis or Jansky-Bielschowsky disease is characterized by an age at onset of 2 to 4 years with mental deterioration and epilepsy, ataxia and loss of eyesight. In the EEG, occipital spike and wave complexes associated with photostimulation, gigantic visual and somatosensory evoked potentials, and disappearance of electroretinographic responses are typical findings. The defective gene is located in chromosome 11p15 and encodes tripeptidyl petidase 1. A Finnish variant of gene error is in chromosome 13q22.

Juvenile form or Spielmeyer-Sjögren disease usually starts with a visual defect followed by increasing learning difficulties, epilepsy and motor problems from the affected extrapyramidal system. The erroneous gene is located in chromosome 16p12 and encodes transmembrane CLN3 protein.

Further forms of neuronal ceroid lipofuscinosis include the late infantile variant of gipsies (chromosome 15q21-23, encoding transmembrane CLN6 protein), Turkish late-infantile variant (chromosome 8p23 in a part of the cases) and Northern epilepsy or epilepsy with progressive mental retardation located in chromosome 8p23.

X-linked LD syndromes

Fragile-X syndrome is the most common monogenic disease with LD. The estimates of incidences are 1 in 1,250 male births and 1 in 2,500 female births. No striking features occur at early age, although gaze avoidance, tactile defensiveness, shyness and autistic-like social withdrawal may be found in boys and girls during early years. From puberty, the triad of LD, typical dysmorphic facies and macroorchidism are very helpful in male patients. The dysmorphisms of the facies include long, narrow face with prominent forehead, prognathia, and large ears. The triad is complemented by high-arched palate, pectus excavatus, mitral valve prolapse, dilatation of ascending aorta, hyperextensible finger joints, flat feet, and plantar and simian creases.

Behaviour is characterised by hyperactivity, stereotypic hand waving and finger biting, gaze avoidance, continuous shyness and autistic traits. Speech is fast, echolalic and poor in contents. Epileptic seizures are common. LD is moderate but may be severe. In magnetic resonance imaging studies of adult male fragile-X patients, virtually all showed cerebral and cerebellar cortical and white matter atrophy (Brunberg et al., 2002). According to knockout mouse experiments, the absence of the FMR protein coded by FMR1 gene impairs maturation and pruning of synapses, notably in the context of experience-dependent development of cortical circuits (Bardoni and Mandel, 2002). The ascertainment of the diagnosis is usually based on the demonstration of an expansion of the trinucleotide repeat flanking the gene FMR1.

Rett's syndrome occurs worldwide in about 1 in 10,000 live born girls. Rett's syndrome starts with a stagnation of motor and mental development at the age of 0.5 to 1.5 years. A rapid destruction stage then follows with peculiar hand wringing or washing movements, and severe mental deterioration with autistic features. The condition ends to motor deterioration and cachexia. Rett's syndrome was long considered lethal in boys, but affected boys have recently been reported. It is caused by mutation of the gene MECP2 encoding methyl-CpG binding protein 2 which functions as a repressor of gene transcription. The mutated gene is unable to silence target genes and inappropriate gene expression leads to the clinical phenotype. The disease has an X-chromosomal dominant inheritance pattern, i.e. affected girls are heterozygous for the MECP2 gene, and the majority of cases are sporadic.

MISCELLANEOUS

There is a large but gradually decreasing number of disorders, where either the pedigree refers to monogenic inheritance or is polygenic with no apparent mode of inheritance. An identification of a specific aetiology will be more probable if the proband and several relatives have LD associated with distinct dysmorphisms and/or malformations. The identification of a genetic factor may be less likely if family data or major dysmorphic features are lacking.

A number of conditions with probable genetic traits exist which have an apparent multifactorial background. These include disorders of dorsal and ventral induction and proliferation of the neuronal tissue during embryonic and foetal periods. In cases of *neural tube defects*, for example, the role of folate is important because of the methylenetetrahydrofolate gene polymorphism. The homozygosity of the mutation ($677C \rightarrow T$) of the gene increases the risk for spina bifida and anencephaly, which can be prevented by folate supplementation (Ou *et al.*, 1996).

Hydrocephalus is a major complication and often associated with LD, particularly in case of many shunt revisions and central nervous system infections.

Holoprosencephaly with a defective formation of the midline of the cerebral hemispheres shows a strong association with the trisomies 13 and 18, but is also associated with abnormalities of several other chromosomes including 2p21, 7q36, 18p and 21q22.3. In their overview, of mutations in holoprosencephaly, Wallis and Muenke (2000) indicated that at least 12 different loci are associated with holoprosencephaly and several distinct genes have been identified. LD is usually severe particularly in patients who have early symptoms such as infantile spasms with hypsarrhythmia.

Disorders of proliferation, such as true megalencephaly and hemimegalencephaly, are often associated with disorders of migration and organization, and exemplify syndromic disorders which probably have a genetic aetiology and are often associated with severe LD.

Disorders of migration with at least partial genetic aetiology and LD include agyria/pachygyria, microgyria, and agenesis of corpus callosum. Type 1 lissencephaly presents with polymicrogyria, pachygyria or agyria or their mixture. Some cases show dominant inheritance (Aicardi, 1991). A small number are caused by deletion of the distal part of chromosome 17p13- being included in Miller-Dieker syndrome (see above). Cobblestone (type II) lissencephaly is found in the Warburg-Walker syndrome which consists of a smooth cerebral cortex, thick meninges, small cerebellum with lack of vermis, absence of pyramidal tracts, severe muscular dystrophy and hydrocephalus in most of the cases. The Walker-Warburg syndrome and muscle-eye-brain disease are distinct disorders; while the muscle-eye-brain gene has been located to chromosome 1p32-p34, the linkage to that locus was excluded in seven of eight Walker-Warburg families (Cormand *et al.*, 2001).

Finally, there is a group of LD disorders with no malformation syndrome, except for possible minor dysmorphisms. This group includes diseases with unknown but suspected genetic aetiologies. One example is infantile autism, where genome scans suggest linkage to chromosomes 7q, 2q, 3q and X (Auranen *et al.*, 2002).

PREVENTION

Prevention is possible in some selected patients with genetic LD. Primary prevention includes screening of carriers, preconceptional genetic counselling, and planning of individual pregnancies. Many ethical questions are associated with these issues, but they are not discussed here.

Screening of the population for the respective disorder is possible if a reasonably reliable laboratory or clinical marker for the disorder is available. Basically, all diseases with a known mode of inheritance and likelihood of mutations can be screened. The cost-benefit calculations, however, must be considered. Recently, a consensus statement on screening and management of phenylketonuria has been given (National Institutes of Health Consensus Development Panel, 2001). Well arranged, antenatal screening is feasible and effective in finding carriers of genetic diseases (Hietala *et al.*, 1996).

One of the aims of genetic counselling is to predict the likelihood of recurrence, i.e. inheriting the disease from a parent or by a new mutation. The recurrence risks in siblings for many diseases are known and show, for example, that the risk LD is 4-5-fold, but in male sibling of a male patient 6-12-fold (Herbst and Baird, 1982). The recurrence risk for all sibs of male index patient with severe LD vary from 3.5% to 14% (Crow and Tolmie, 1998). The counselling starts with a careful previous history with assessment of the family pedigree. In case of maternal epilepsy and risk of offspring LD, for example, planning of an individual pregnancy means developing as optimal circumstances as possible, with adjustment of external factors such as the mother's eventual medication and assessment of possible needs for preventive drug therapy like folate. Folate supplementation has proved beneficial in the overall prevention of neural tube defects. (Green, 2002).

Secondary prevention aims at as early as possible detection of any problems since the first trimester to the latest expected age of onset of the disorder. During the first trimester, ultrasound examination, determination of amnion fluid alpha-fetoprotein and chromosomal analysis may detect an affected foetus. A typical example is Down syndrome in expectant mothers of advancing age. A pre-implantation genetic diagnosis excludes the necessity of a therapeutic abortion (Grifo *et al.*, 1998). Prenatal gene therapy for severe genetic developmental disorders is now feasible but, among other things, raises concerns about inducing mutagenesis and subsequent tumour formation (Ye *et al.*, 2001).

The second and third trimester examinations include regular visits to maternity health units to check and advise on life-style and the conditions under which the person lives, check-ups of blood drug concentrations if needed, and cardio topographic and ultrasound examinations for malformations, intrauterine growth retardation, or signs of asphyxia.

Tertiary prevention intends to minimise the consequences of the disorder after its onset. In addition to an antiepileptic drug therapy for patients with epilepsy, various medications have been found beneficial in different diseases with LD. These include tetrahydrobiopterin against disabling depression and panic attacks in mild phenylalaninaemia (Koch *et al.*, 2002), topiramate against self-injurious behaviour in Prader-Willi syndrome (Shapira *et al.*, 2002), and levodopa, baclofen and tizanidine against extrapyramidal symptoms and myoclonia in juvenile neuronal ceroid lipofuscinosis. Qualitative and quantitative dietary arrangements have been applied, for example, to phenylketonuria and Prader-Willi syndrome. Intractable epilepsy and LD in megalencephaly and similar conditions may be amenable to surgical treatment. Bone marrow transplantation therapy may initially decrease excretion into urine of some degradation products in aspartylglucosaminuria, but in a long run no clinical effect can be demonstrated. Gene therapy may become included in this therapeutic process in future.

CONCLUSION

Specific genetic aetiologies for many LDs are being discovered and multiple loci responsible for polygenic traits are being unravelled increasingly, as a result of the rapid progress in the human genome project. The speed of novel methods and techniques will probably be accelerating and help understanding of the genetic aetiology and pathogenesis of diseases and the interactions of genetic factors with environmental effects. In recent years too, large steps have been taken in the prevention of genetic diseases causing LD.

REFERENCES

Aicardi, J. (1991). The agygyria / pachygyria complex: a spectrum of cortical malformations. *Brain and Devel* **13**, 1-8.

Åkesson, H.O. (1986). The biological origin of mild mental retardation. A critical view. *Acta Psychiat Scand* **13**, 1-8.

Arvio, M. and Sillanpää, M. (2003). Prevalence, aetiology and comorbidity of severe and profound intellectual disability in Finland. *J Intellect Disabil Res* **47**(2), 108-112.

Auranen, M., Vanhala, R., Varilo, T., Ayers, K., Kempas, E., Ylisaukko-oja, T., Sinsheimer, JS., Peltonen L., and Järvelä, I. (2002). A genome-wide screen for autism spectrum disorders: evidence for a major susceptibility locus on chromosome 3q25-27. *Am J Hum Genet* **71**, 777-790.

Bardoni, B. and Mandel, J.L. (2002). Advances in understanding of fragile X pathogenesis and FMRP function, and in identification of X linked mental retardation genes. *Curr Opin Genet Dev* **12**, 284-293.

Bienvenu, T., Poirier, K., Friocourt, G., Bahi, N., Beaumont, D. et al. (2002). ARX, a novel Prd-class-homeobox gene highly expressed in the telencephalon, is mutated in X-linked mental retardation. *Hum Mol Genet* **11**, 981-991.

Bond, J., Roberts, E., Mochida, G.H., Hampshire, D.J., Scott, S., Askham, J.M. et al. (2002). ASPM is a major determinant of cerebral cortical size. *Nat Gene* **32**, 316-320.

Brunberg, J.A., Jacquemont, S., Hagerman, R.J., Berry-Kravis, E.M., Grigsby, J., Leehey, M.A., Tassone, F., Brown, W.T., Greco, C.M. and Hagerman, P.J. (2002). Fragile-X premutation carriers: characteristic MR imaging findings of adult male patients with progressive cerebellar and cognitive dysfunction. *Am J Neuroradiol* **23**, 1757-1766.

Cantani, A. and Gagliesi, D. (1998). Rubinstein-Taybi syndrome. Review of 732 cases and analysis of the typical traits. *Eur Rev Med Pharmacol Sci* **2**, 81-87.

Clarkson, B., Pavenski, K., Dupuis, L., Kennedy, S., Meyn, S., Nezarati, M.M., Nie, G., Weksberg, R., Withers, S., Quercia, N., Teebi, A.S. and Teshima, I. (2002). Detecting rearrangements in children using subtelomeric FISH and SKY. *Am J Med Genet* **107**, 267-274.

Cormand, B., Pihko H., Bayes, M., Valanne, L., Santavuori, P., Talim, B et al. (2001). Clinical and genetic distinction between Walker-Warburg syndrome and muscle-eye-brain disease. *Neurol* **56**, 1059-1069.

Crow, Y.J. and Tolmie, J.L. (1998). Recurrence risks in mental retardation. *J Med Genet* **35**, 177-182.

de Vries, B.B., Mohkamsing, S., van den Ouweland, A.M., Halley, D.J., Niermeijer, M.F., Oostra, B.A. and Willemsen, R. (1998). Screening with the FMR1 protein test among mentally retarded males. *Hum Genet* **103**, 520-522.

Down, J.L.H. (1866). Observations on an ethnic classification of idiots. *London Hospital Reports* **3**, 259-265.

Eronen, M., Peippo, M., Hiippala, A., Raatikka, M., Arvio, M., Johansson, R. and Kähkönen, M. (2002). Cardiovascular manifestations in 75 patients with Williams syndrome. *J Med Genet* **39**, 554-558.

Fryers, T. (1984). *The epidemiology of severe intellectual impairment. The dynamics of prevalence.* Academic Press, London.

Galvan Manso, M., Campistol, J., Monros, E., Poo, P., Vernet, A.M., Pineda, M., Sans, A., Colomer, J., Conill, J.J. and Sanmarti, F.X. (2002). Angelman syndrome: physical characteristics and behavioural phenotype in 37 patients with confirmed genetic diagnosis. *Revista de Neurologia* **35**, 425-429. (In Spanish).

Green, N.S. (2002). Folic acid supplementation and prevention of birth defects. *J Nutr* **132**(suppl.), 2356-2360.

Grifo, J.A., Giatras, K., Tang, Y.X. and Krey, L.C. (1998). Successful outcome with day 4 embryo transfer after preimplantation diagnosis for genetically transmitted diseases. *Hum Reprod* **13**, 1656-1659.

Herbst, D.S. and Baird, P.A. (1982). Sib risks for nonspecific mental retardation in British Columbia. *Am J Med Genet* **13**, 197-208.

Hietala, M., Aula, P., Syvanen, A.C., Isoniemi, A., Peltonen, L., and Palotie, A. (1996). DNA-based carrier screening in primary healthcare: screening for aspartylglucosaminuria mutations in maternity health offices. *Clin Chem* **42**, 1398-1404.

Hou, J.W., Wang, T.R. and Chuang, S.M. (1998). An epidemiological and aetiological study of children with intellectual disability in Taiwan. *J Intellect Disabil Res* **42**, 137-143.

Koch, R., Guttler, F. and Blau, N. (2002). Mental illness in mild PKU responds to biopterin. *Mol Genet Metab* **75**, 284-286.

Kurotaki, N., Imaizumi, K., Harada, N., Masuno, M., Kondoh, T., Nagai, T. *et al.* (2002). Haploinsufficiency of NSD1 causes Sotos syndrome. *Nat Genet* **4**, 365-366.

Lee, P.D. (2002). Disease management of Prader-Willi syndrome. *Expert Opin Pharmacother* **10**, 1451-1459.

Lejeune, J., Gautier, M. and Turpin, R. (1959). Etudes des chromosomes somatiques de neuf enfants mongoliens. *Comptes Rendus Hebdomadaires des Séances de l'Academie des Sciences* **248**, 1721.

Matilainen, R., Airaksinen, E., Mononen, T., Launiala, K. and Kääriäinen, R. (1995). A population-based study on the causes of mild and severe mental retardation. *Acta Paediatrica* **84**, 261-266.

Mirisola, M.G., Cali, F., Gloria, A., Schinocca, P., D'Amato, M., Cassara, G., Leo, G.D., Palillo, I., Meli, C. and Romano, V. (2001). PAH gene mutations in the Sicilian population: association with mini-haplotypes and expression analysis. *Mol Genet Metab* **74**, 353-361.

National Institutes of Health Consensus Development Panel. (2001). National Institutes of Health consensus development conference statement: phenylketonuria: screening and management. *Pediatrics* **108**, 972-982.

Ou, C.Y., Stevenson, R.E., Brown, V.K., Schwartz, C.E., Allen, W.P., Khoury, M.J., Rozen, R., Oakley, G.P. Jr. and Adams, M.J. Jr. (1996). 5,10 Methylenetetra-hydrofolate reductases genetic polymorphism as a risk factor for neural tube defects. *Am J Med Genet* **63**, 610-614.

Pollack, M.A., Golden, G.S., Schmidt, R., Davis, J.A. and Leeds, N. (1978). Infantile spasms in Down syndrome: a report of 5 cases and review of the literature. *Ann Neurol* **3**, 406-408.

Roberts, P.S., Chung, J., Jozwiak, S., Dabora, S.L., Franz, D.N., Thiele, E.A. and Kwiatkowski, D.J. (2002). SNP identification, haplotype analysis, and parental origin of mutations in TSC2. *Hum Genet* **111**, 96-101.

Shapira, N.A., Lessing, M.C., Murphy, T.K., Driscoll, D.J. and Goodman, W.K. (2002). Topiramate attenuates self-injurious behaviour in Prader –Willi syndrome. *Int J Neuropsychopharmacol* **5**, 141-145.

Steffenberg, U., Hagberg, G. and Kyllerman, M. (1995). Active epilepsy in mentally retarded children. II. Etiology and reduced pre- and perinatal optimality. *Acta Paediatrica* **84**, 1153-1159.

Stromme, P. (2000). Aetiology in severe and mild mental retardation: a population-based study of Norwegian children. *Dev Med Child Neurol* **42**, 76-86.

Stromme, P., Bjornstad, P.G. and Ramstad, K. (2002). Prevalence estimation of Williams syndrome. *J Child Neurol* **17**, 269-271.

Taine, L., Goizet, G., Wen, Z.Q., Petrij, F., Breuning, M.H., Ayme, S., Saura, R., Arveiler, B. and Lacombe, D. (1998). Submicroscopic deletion of chromosome 16p13.3 in patients with Rubinstein-Taybi syndrome. *Am J Med Genet* **78,** 267-270.

Van Buggenhout, G.J., Trijbels, J.M., Wevers, R., Trommelen, J.C., Hamel, B.C., Brunner, H.G. and Fryns, J.P. (2001). Metabolic studies in older mentally retarded patients: significance of metabolic testing and correlation with the clinical phenotype. *Genet Couns* **12**, 1-21.

Wallis, D. and Muenke, M. (2000). Mutations in holoprosencephaly. *Hum Mutat* **16**, 99-108.

Ye, X., Mitchell, M., Newman, K. and Batshaw, M.L. (2001). Prospects for prenatal gene therapy in disorders causing mental retardation. *Ment Retard Dev Disabil Res Rev* **7**, 65-72.

Zoller, M., Rembeck, B., Åkesson, H.O. and Angervall, L. (1995). Life expectancy, mortality and prognostic factors in neurofibromatosis type 1. A twelve-year follow-up of an epidemiological study in Göteborg, Sweden. *Acta Derm Venereol* **75**, 136-140.

Learning Disability and Epilepsy: an Integrative Approach
Edited by Michael R. Trimble
© 2003 Clarius Press Ltd

4

Aetiology of Epilepsy and Learning Disorders: Specific Epilepsy Syndromes; Genetic, Chromosomal and Sporadic Syndromes

RICHARD APPLETON

*Royal Liverpool Children's NHS Trust
Alder Hey, Eaton Road, Liverpool, UK*

INTRODUCTION

Epilepsy is not, and never has been, a single disorder. More appropriately it is a group of disorders or 'epilepsy syndromes', most of which have an onset in childhood, usually developing between the age of six months and twelve years. Many of these syndromes are benign and are not recognized to be accompanied by developmental delay or learning difficulties whereas others are most malignant (sometimes called catastrophic) and are frequently associated with significant learning difficulties. The handicap that accompanies these syndromes may be present at the onset of the seizures or, more commonly, develop as the syndrome evolves including at times of acute and often prolonged exacerbation (eg. episodes of non-convulsive status epilepticus).

Many of these more malignant epilepsy syndromes that are associated with learning disability are not unreasonably termed 'epileptic encephalopathies' in which any cognitive impairment or mental handicap is considered to be directly related not only to the frequency of the clinical seizures, but also to the very frequent, if not at times persistent abnormal inter-ictal (also called sub-clinical) paroxysmal (also called epileptiform) activity recorded on an EEG.

Another potential - and important - cause of the learning difficulties is obviously the aetiology of the epilepsy syndrome. It is important to appreciate that the identification of an epilepsy syndrome does not imply a specific cause and that an individual epilepsy syndrome may arise from different causes. Many will be found to have a defined cause (ie: symptomatic), having arisen as a consequence of an early brain injury (eg: meningo-encephalitis, trauma or severe hypoxia or ischaemia) or as part of a chromosomal disorder (eg: Down's syndrome, or ring chromosome 20) or a genetic syndrome (eg: Aicardi, Angelman and Rett syndromes). However, a significant number of the syndromes or epileptic encephalopathies are cryptogenic or idiopathic, with no identified underlying cause.

The objective of this Chapter is to briefly describe those epilepsy syndromes or epileptic encephalopathies that are known to be associated with severe learning difficulties. The Chapter will also discuss some of the more common chromosomal disorders or genetic syndromes and sporadic diseases that are frequently characterized by both epilepsy and severe learning difficulties. (Aicardi, 1998; Roger, et al., 1992; Singh et al., 2002). The relationship between learning difficulties and inter-ictal (sub-clinical) paroxysmal (epileptiform) activity will be discussed in Chapter 8.

EPILEPSY SYNDROMES

Epileptic encephalopathy with burst-suppression (early neonatal and early infantile myoclonic encephalopathy including Ohtahara syndrome).

Epileptic encephalopathies with burst-suppression on the electroencephalogram (EEG) may present in the first few weeks or months of life with multiple seizure types, both focal and generalized and including myoclonus. The development of brief tonic, and also commonly, partial seizures, between one and four months of age, together with burst-suppression on EEG is often termed Ohtahara syndrome (Yamatogi and Ohtahara, 2002). Even with the early age of onset of these frequent seizures, there may already be clear evidence of developmental delay and this certainly becomes more obvious and more profound as these encephalopathies develop and evolve during the first year of life. The precise cause of the developmental delay and cognitive impairment is unclear but probably represents a combination of the underlying cause of the encephalopathy together with frequent seizures (often occurring up to more than 100 times a day) and very frequent, if not continuous inter-ictal (sub-clinical) epileptiform activity.

A number of conditions may be associated with these early neonatal and early infantile encephalopathies including cerebral dysgenesis (specifically, lissencephaly and schizencephaly – for further details see Chapter 5), Aicardi syndrome, Rett syndrome (commonly, but not exclusively in male neonates with this condition) and a number of metabolic conditions (specifically, non-ketotic hyperglycinaemia, methylmalonic/proprionic acidaemia, pyridoxine deficiency, biotinidase deficiency and Menkes disease). However, in most children who present with either early neonatal or early infantile epileptic encephalopathy, no obvious structural or metabolic cause is identified.

The prognosis of these different encephalopathies is universally poor, irrespective of the underlying cause. Those children who survive into the second half of the first year of life frequently develop West syndrome and many children do not reach their second or third birthday. Survivors are usually left with refractory epilepsy, spastic tetraplegia, cortical visual impairment and severe mental handicap.

Migrating partial seizures in infancy

This is another rare epilepsy syndrome, having an onset in the first six months of life (Coppola, *et al.*, 1995). The initial and predominant seizure type is partial (focal) often with significant autonomic features. Towards the end of the second half of the first year of life (six to 12 months of age), the seizure frequency increases and on EEG, the seizures can be shown to arise from different areas of the cortex – which is why the term 'migrating' is ascribed to this epilepsy syndrome. Coincidental with this increase in seizure frequency towards the end of the first year of life, there is marked developmental slowing followed by a plateau in the child's development if not some regression. Simultaneous video-EEG telemetry may demonstrate a clear correlation between the anatomical site or topography of the EEG ictal discharge and the clinical features of the seizure (eg: occipitally-sited EEG seizures occur in association with lateral deviation of the head and eyes and lateral eye jerks, while temporally-sited EEG seizures are commonly associated with staring, automatisms and repetitive chewing movements).

Most children have normal brain imaging and metabolic studies, and the frequent and repeated seizures, including episodes of both complex partial and generalized convulsive status epilepticus are resistant to all anti-epileptic medication, including corticosteroids.

The long-term prognosis is poor including death, severe developmental delay or learning difficulties and the frequent evolution of both microcephaly and involuntary movements.

West Syndrome

The association of infantile spasms and EEG findings of hypsarrhythmia define the syndrome that Dr. West described so explicitly in his own son in 1841 (West, 1841; Wong and Trevathan 2001). Children may present from one to 13 or 14 months of age, although the peak age is between six and nine months. The developmental delay and cognitive impairment that commonly evolves and is ultimately found in over 75-80% of affected patients, is not essential for the diagnosis of West syndrome. The cognitive impairment and subsequent mental handicap are predominantly related to the underlying cause although it is possible that the control of both the spasms and resolution of the hypsarrhythmia may also contribute to the long-term developmental and intellectual outcome. This may be particularly relevant to tuberous sclerosis (TS), a neurocutaneous disorder and one of the more common causes of West syndrome. Prior to the introduction of the anti-epileptic drug vigabatrin, the long-term intellectual/cognitive prognosis of children with TS presenting with infantile spasms was almost universally poor; the often dramatic response of both the spasms and resolution of the hypsarrhythmia following treatment with vigabatrin appears to correlate closely with the improved cognitive status of these children with this disorder (Chiron, et al., 1997).

Unfortunately, approximately 65% of children with West syndrome will develop more chronic epilepsy, including the Lennox-Gastaut syndrome, which itself is characterized by severe learning difficulties.

Additional specific causes of West syndrome, including cerebral malformations (eg: lissencephaly and polymicrogyria) and as a sequel to perinatal hypoxic-ischaemic encephalopathy, are typically associated with a very poor long-term outlook with regard to both the development of chronic and drug-resistant epilepsy and also severe learning difficulties. Again, this reflects predominantly the underlying cause rather than its treatment or the response to treatment (Appleton, 2001; Riikonen, 2001).

Severe myoclonic epilepsy in infancy

Severe myoclonic epilepsy in infancy is fortunately a rare syndrome that has a very poor prognosis in terms of seizure-control and mental development (Roger, et al., 1992; Kanazawa, 2001). Seizure onset is usually between three and nine months of age with what initially are considered to be febrile seizures that are prolonged and may either be unilateral or generalized. If EEGs are undertaken within the first year of life, the findings are usually normal. By 18-24 months of age there is typically an explosive onset of unilateral clonic or generalized tonic-clonic seizures without any triggering or provoking febrile illness. Frequent myoclonic seizures develop from the end of the second year of life and may persist for many years. Tonic-clonic and myoclonic status are also common and tend to persist despite the use of benzodiazepines (administered either as 'rescue' or long-term maintenance medication) and other, conventional anti-epileptic drugs. Although EEGs may initially be normal in the first year of life, by the age of two or three years, marked abnormalities are seen, including generalized polyspike and slow wave or slow, spike and slow wave activity which may be prolonged and consistent with episodes of electrical or non-convulsive status epilepticus. Frequent myoclonic and clonic seizures may be focal (flitting from one part of the body to the other) or generalized, and partial seizures may also occur. Perhaps not surprisingly in view of the multiple seizure types and overall clinical picture, this epilepsy syndrome is sometimes known as severe polymorphous epilepsy of infancy.

There is often a strong family history of epilepsy in children with severe myoclonic epilepsy in infancy – including febrile seizures (without later epilepsy) and generalized tonic-clonic seizures. At the current time severe myoclonic epilepsy in infancy is considered to be just one of the many clinical phenotypes within the genetic syndrome of generalized epilepsy and febrile seizures 'plus' (Scheffer and Berkovic, 1997; Singh, et al., 1999; Singh, et al., 2001).

Early development is usually normal although the situation usually changes dramatically by the end of the second year of life. Although subsequent developmental delay may be global there is a particular prediliction for speech and language difficulties. Unfortunately, the long-term prognosis of this syndrome is poor both with regard to persisting and often drug-resistant clonic and tonic-clonic seizures but also with regard to cognitive and educational impairment. Most children develop severe learning difficulties and not surprisingly require special schooling, notably within schools that incorporate specialized language units.

Myoclonic epilepsy in non-progressive and progressive myoclonic epilepsies.

Myoclonic seizures are a common seizure type in a large number of both non-progressive but also progressive myoclonic epilepsies (Aicardi, 1998). Atonic and tonic-clonic seizures are additional seizure types in many of these different epilepsies and episodes of both convulsive (tonic-clonic but also myoclonic) and non-convulsive (absence) status epilepticus are common. Examples of non-progressive myoclonic epilepsies include sequelae to diffuse and usually severe cerebral insults (eg: hypoxia, trauma, encephalitis) and as a component of a number of genetic syndromes (eg: Angelman). In addition, there are a large number of disorders that may present as progressive myoclonic epilepsy (Table 1), some of which are described later in this Chapter. The cognitive difficulties and often severe mental handicap that usually develop in these children reflect both the inherent cerebral (cortical) component of the condition (whether acquired or genetic) as well as a consequence of frequent seizures and episodes of status epilepticus.

Table 1.   Progressive myoclonic epilepsies.

Neuronal ceroid lipofuscinoses

       acute infantile

       late infantile

Infantile hexosaminidase deficiency

       Tay-Sachs disease

       Sandhoff's disease

Sialidosis Type 1 (cherry red spot-myoclonus syndrome)

Sialidosis Type 2

Mucolipidosis Type 1

Myoclonic epilepsy with ragged-red fibres (MERRF)

       (a mitochondrial cytopathy)

Juvenile Huntington's disease

Lafora body disease

Unverricht-Lundborg disease

Landau-Kleffner syndrome

First described in 1957, this rare disorder is also known as 'a syndrome of acquired aphasia with convulsive disorder', or 'acquired epileptic aphasia' or 'acquired aphasia of childhood with epilepsy', based on clear clinical and EEG criteria (Kolski and Otsubo, 2002). There is also an overlap with another epilepsy syndrome of 'continuous spike-wave in slow sleep' which is also known as 'electrical status epilepticus of slow sleep'. Over 50% of patients present between the ages of three and eight years with verbal agnosia (severe impairment or loss of verbal and auditory understanding) and expressive aphasia. The remaining 50% of children present initially with epileptic seizures and an additional 20-30% of children develop seizures some weeks or months after the onset of the verbal agnosia and expressive aphasia. The seizures may be multiple but usually include complex partial (with focal motor and atypical absence symptomatology), generalized tonic-clonic and atonic ('drop') seizures. Nocturnal seizures and episodes of both convulsive and non-convulsive status epilepticus are common. During wakefulness, the EEG typically shows multi-focal slow, spike and spike-wave discharges in either the temporal or centro-temporal regions. During sleep the EEG shows more dramatic changes with bursts of prolonged slow, spike-slow wave discharges which may be either focal or more commonly generalized and may last for many minutes (possibly hours), and it is this specific finding that is shared with the syndrome of continuous spike-waves in slow sleep. This is discussed further by Besag (Chapter 7).

Behavioural disturbances are also common and may not simply arise as a secondary, and often 'frustrating' complication to the verbal agnosia and expressive aphasia, but may reflect the very frequent abnormal inter-ictal EEG activity particularly during sleep. An additional cause of the behavioural (and language) difficulties may also be the underlying aetiology, although as yet, none have yet been identified in this syndrome.

Children with Landau-Kleffner syndrome (LKS) are not infrequently misdiagnosed initially as being deaf or having a primary conduct disorder. Although non-verbal cognitive functioning may be normal at presentation, more global intellectual impairment may be seen if the syndrome is diagnosed late or the response to treatment is particularly poor.

Seizure control in LKS is achieved relatively easily with conventional anti-epileptic drugs (including sodium valproate, clobazam and rarely vigabatrin), and the seizures tend to remit spontaneously by the age of 15 or 16 years. In contrast, the verbal agnosia and receptive and expressive speech difficulties and behavioural problems may persist despite optimal medical treatment. Currently, the usual therapeutic approach is with sodium valproate either used as monotherapy or in combination with prednisolone, the latter used in low dose for a number of months. Subpial transection may be a useful surgical therapeutic option but the data are limited and would suggest that the beneficial effects are seen only if the procedure is undertaken within two or three years of presentation (Robinson, et al., 2001).

Lennox-Gastaut syndrome

This is one of the more common, but still over-diagnosed malignant (catastrophic) epilepsy syndromes that is characterized by multiple seizure types and characteristic EEG findings and almost invariably, learning difficulties which are usually severe (Roger, et al., 1992; Crumrine, 2002; Niedermeyer, 2002). The age of onset of Lennox-Gastaut syndrome (LGS) is between one and ten years of age, although the peak age of onset is between two and six years. The earlier the onset the more likely an underlying cause will be found. Approximately one third of children will develop LGS having initially had West syndrome in the first year of life. Cryptogenic cases – where no cause is identified – are common and tend to have a slightly later age of onset (between five and eight years of age). Symptomatic cases may be caused by focal, multifocal or diffuse cerebral insults that may be both acquired and congenital (including as part of specific genetic or chromosomal disorders).

The characteristic or defining seizure type in LGS is tonic, usually of the trunk and most commonly during sleep. Prolonged atypical absence, atonic and clonic-tonic seizures are also common. Complex partial and myoclonic seizures are seen infrequently and if myoclonic seizures dominate the clinical picture, the diagnosis is unlikely to be LGS and would suggest more the possibility of either myoclonic-astatic epilepsy or an evolving progressive myoclonic epilepsy. Children frequently experience episodes of both convulsive but also importantly, non-convulsive status epilepticus, both of which may contribute to the severe learning difficulties that are eventually seen in over 90% of patients.

Inter-ictal EEG findings comprise of frequent paroxysms of slow, spike and slow wave activity occurring with a frequency of 1-2 Hz and fast spiking activity (10-14 Hz) seen during tonic seizures. Episodes of non-convulsive status (manifest by atypical absence with hypersalivation and some motor features) are also common and may be difficult to recognize, particularly in view of the fact that these children have severe learning and behavioural difficulties. It is important to listen to the parents and other carers of these children as they are likely to be the first to identify that their child may be in non-convulsive status – through a change in the child's behaviour (becoming unusually quiet or withdrawn when usually they are very hyperactive) with or without motor features including subtle myoclonus and excessive drooling. The EEG is clearly important in confirming or excluding non-convulsive status.

Most children will show evidence of developmental delay or learning difficulties at the onset of LGS, particularly if they have previously had West syndrome or other seizure types in the first year of life. Initially these difficulties may be mild or moderate. However, by late childhood and adolescence over 90% of patients will demonstrate severe learning difficulties. The evolution of these frequently encompasses some early regression - or loss of skills - in most areas but particularly in communication and gross motor function. Many children also develop evidence of frontal lobe dysfunction as manifest by a very limited attention span, poor judgment, no sense of danger, impulsivity and grossly disinhibited verbal and physical behaviour.

A number of factors may contribute to the progressive handicap that is seen in patients with LGS. The contribution of each of these individual factors is difficult, if not impossible to determine, but would include the following:

- frequent and drug-resistant clinical seizures;

- frequent and potentially unrecognized episodes of non-convulsive (atypical absence) status epilepticus;

- frequent, if not continuous (during sleep) slow, spike and slow wave activity even in the absence of clinical seizures;

- the underlying cause of the syndrome;

- the cumulative effects of repeated head injuries sustained during the tonic and atonic seizures that characterize this syndrome;

- the effect of the simultaneous use of multiple anti-epileptic drugs – and often in high doses – to try and control the seizures.

Although there is a significant mortality in patients with LGS, most survive and by adolescence, although the seizures may be less frequent and are usually confined to tonic-clonic seizures, are left with severe learning difficulties and are fully dependent on others to meet their daily needs.

SPECIFIC SYNDROMES (GENETIC AND CHROMOSOMAL) FEATURING EPILEPSY AND SEVERE LEARNING DIFFICULTIES OR MENTAL HANDICAP.

Pyridoxine deficiency

This autosomal recessive disorder is rare but because it is largely treatable, the diagnosis should not be overlooked. Children usually present within the few days after birth with frequent and different seizure types (specifically myoclonic, tonic and clonic) but onset may be in utero or as late as 12-18 months of age. Infants are generally irritable and hypertonic. The EEG is markedly abnormal showing multifocal discharges, a burst-suppression pattern or modified (atypical) hypsarrythmia. Occasionally the seizures may show a partial response to conventional antiepileptic drugs (AEDs) – which may delay making the diagnosis. More commonly, the seizures are very frequent and are resistant to all AEDs but respond dramatically to pyridoxine. Clinical response to intravenous pyridoxine is usually immediate, as is normalization of the EEG, although the latter may be delayed for days or weeks.

In equivocal cases a trial of pyridoxine should be given for at least four or even six weeks and any infant under the age of 18 months with intractable seizures (particularly if no cause for the seizures has been identified) should receive a trial of the drug. Learning difficulties are common, particularly if the diagnosis is established late and tend to be irreversible, even if pyridoxine is then prescribed. Conversely, early diagnosis and treatment with pyridoxine may be associated with near normal or occasionally normal cognitive function (Baxter, *et al.*, 1996).

Aicardi syndrome

This is a rare and possibly X-linked dominantly-inherited condition, affecting predominantly girls, that presents in the first few weeks or months of life with partial and generalized (myoclonic and tonic-clonic) seizures, that frequently evolves into West syndrome with early-onset infantile spasms (Aicardi, 1998). All seizures, including spasms are resistant to medication. Characteristic retinal lesions (choroidal lacunae – large, irregular, 'punched-out' lesions) with or without coloboma of the optic disc are an invariable finding and their absence precludes the diagnosis of Aicardi syndrome. Cerebral malformations are common – typically including agenesis or dysgenesis of the corpus callosum - but also including periventricular heterotopia, ependymal cysts and holoprosencephaly – and vertebrocostal abnormalities are found in approximately 50% of cases. Developmental progress is extremely limited and severe mental handicap is common; children also develop a spastic tetraplegia and microcephaly. Many girls do not survive childhood. No specific genetic defect or chromosomal abnormality has yet been identified in Aicardi syndrome.

Cerebral agyria (lissencephaly) and polymicrogyria/pachygyria

A number of fascinating syndromes – many genetically-determined – have been identified that are of early-onset (neonatal period or infancy), and present with drug-resistant seizures, severe developmental delay and learning difficulties and varying types of neuronal migration abnormalities that are identified on magnetic resonance imaging (MRI) (Clark, 2001; Guerrini and Carrozzo, 2001; Crino, et al., 2002; Pilz, et al., 2002). Many of these children are microcephalic and have dysmorphic facial features (eg: Miller-Dieker syndrome – narrow, pointed forehead, long philtrum, upturned nares, digital abnormalities, lissencephaly ['smooth brain'] on MRI and a deletion of chromosome 17p 13.3 including the lissencephaly 1 gene identified by fluorescent in situ hybridization [FISH]).

Mitochondrial cytopathies (and other metabolic disorders)

A number of mitochondrial cytopathies have been identified that may either present with or feature epilepsy (often myoclonic seizures) and learning difficulties – the latter often progressive (Aicardi, 1998; Lyon, et al., 1996; Gropman, 2001). The 'original' mitochondrial cytopathy that typically featured epilepsy (specifically myoclonic epilepsy) was 'MERRF', an acronym for **M**yoclonic **E**pilepsy and **R**agged **R**ed **F**ibres (the ragged red fibres identified on muscle biopsy). However, it has become clear that other mitochondrial cytopathies may also cause severe epilepsy including Leigh's syndrome and specific enzyme deficiencies (eg: cytochrome oxidase deficiency, pyruvate dehydrogenase deficiency, guanidine-acetate methyl transferase [GAMT] deficiency). The clinical phenotype or spectrum of the mitochondrial cytopathies is very large (and still expanding), and includes muscle weakness, ataxia, retinal pigmentation, ophthalmoplegia, sensorineural deafness, cardiomyopathy and growth retardation. Presentation may be at any age, but commonly is in infancy and early childhood and with variable prognoses, depending on the specific metabolic defect. Early clues to a possible mitochondrial disorder include raised lactate levels in the blood and particularly in the cerebrospinal fluid (CSF) and MRI findings (symmetrical abnormalities within the basal ganglia and brain stem). The diagnosis of a mitochondrial disorder can be confirmed either by DNA analysis (typically on blood or muscle) – although this is only possible for those disorders in which mutations have been identified – or by measuring the activities of individual mitochondrial respiratory chain enzymes in muscle.

There are a large number of other metabolic disorders that may present with or feature a combination of epilepsy and learning difficulties that are outside the remit of this chapter (Aicardi, 1998; Lyon, *et al.*, 1996).

Angelman syndrome

Previously known as the 'happy puppet syndrome', this is an uncommon, but probably under-diagnosed genetic disorder that presents within the first year of life with developmental delay, which though global, eventually has a predilection for speech and language skills – to the extent that these children may develop no meaningful expressive speech (Laan, *et al.*, 1999; Williams, *et al.*, 2001). The abnormal 'jerky' movements, ataxia and frequent myoclonus become obvious during the second year of life and ultimately almost 90% of children will develop epileptic seizures which though very frequent, are usually brief (atypical absences, tonic and atonic but infrequent tonic-clonic in type). Another very common characteristic feature of the syndrome is the frequent and unprovoked bursts of laughter in association with an almost persistently happy disposition; this laughter can be very infectious! The children also have subtle dysmorphic features and may demonstrate autistic features and stereotypic hand movements – features that may closely resemble Rett syndrome. Children with Angelman syndrome usually have severe and some are almost ineducable. The EEG shows runs of spike and slow wave activity with a frequency of 2-3 Hz, predominantly in the anterior regions but also posteriorly, particularly on passive eye closure. Neuroimaging is usually normal. Approximately 75% of patients will be found to have deletions or re-arrangements in the long arm of chromosome 15 (15q 11-13) with the deletion always being on the maternal arm of chromosome 15 (a similar deletion on the paternal chromosome 15 results in a completely different clinical phenotype – the Prader-Willi syndrome, which is not usually associated with epilepsy).

Rett syndrome

Another uncommon but also certainly under-diagnosed genetic disorder occurring in 1 in 10-15,000 girls with a clinical phenotype that is wider than originally thought and now includes boys (Dunn and MacLeod, 2001; Jan *et al.*, 1999). In girls, presentation is typically within the first six to 15 months of life with developmental plateau, truncal hypotonia, early autistic features and deceleration in head growth, ultimately leading to microcephaly by two to four years of age. From one to three years there is then a more explosive (also called 'destructive') phase characterized by regression (specifically loss of any previously acquired language), irritability, loss of purposeful hand movements and characteristic hand stereotypies that tend to be in the child's midline ('hand-wringing', hand-washing, hand-clasping / clapping). Seizures may also develop and are commonly multiple including complex partial, atypical absence and tonic-clonic. Respiratory and autonomic disturbances also develop often after the age of three years but sometimes as early as 15-18 months of age – and are manifest by periods of shallow breathing, hyperventilation and apnoea that may be prolonged, resulting in peri-oral cyanosis and syncope that may be misdiagnosed as epileptic seizures.

Approximately 75% of children never walk independently and those that do often lose the ability after the age of 10 or 12 years. This motor deterioration is frequently accompanied by the development of a kyphoscoliosis and trophic changes to the hands and feet, including acrocyanosis. In contrast, seizure frequency tends to diminish in late childhood or early adolescence. The majority (> 90%) of children will be handicapped and this is usually severe. Life expectancy may be reduced, particularly in those patients who have never learnt to walk or who have severe epilepsy.

The EEG may be useful in establishing the diagnosis – with different abnormalities at the different stages of the disorder and neuroimaging is normal. Fortunately, the recent identification of the common DNA mutation in the methyl-CpG binding protein 2 (MeCP2), gene has made the diagnostic process much easier. However, the identification of this mutation in male infants who presented with a severe epileptic encephalopathy (some of whom subsequently died in late infancy) and also in older boys with an almost identical pattern to that seen in girls has clearly demonstrated that there is a far broader clinical phenotype than previously thought and as originally described by Professor Andreas Rett in Austria in 1966. At present, approximately 80% of girls with the 'classical' Rett syndrome phenotype will be found to have a mutation in the MeCP2 gene on chromosome Xq28; it is possible that the remaining 20% may have a different abnormality (eg: a gross deletion) within the gene.

Late infantile neuronal ceroid lipofuscinosis (Jansky-Bielschowsky disease)

This is a autosomal recessive disorder that, after usually normal development, presents at between two and four years of age with myoclonic and tonic-clonic seizures (Aicardi, 1998; Lyon, *et al.*, 1996). Within 12 months of the onset, irregular asymmetric myoclonus (polymyoclonia) develops that may be induced by proprioceptive stimuli or sudden movements. This is then followed by ataxia, which is due to a combination of frequent polymyoclonia and cerebellar involvement. Within two or three years of presentation children develop a marked ataxic dysarthria, visual impairment (cortical and retinal in origin, the latter due to macular degeneration and consequent optic atrophy) and progressive cognitive impairment. Not uncommonly children are initially diagnosed as having idiopathic epilepsy and the early, mild ataxia is often ascribed to the side-effects of medication (sodium valproate, clonazepam) used to treat the seizures. Most children lose the ability to walk by six or seven years of age, and are severely learning disabled by seven or eight and die by between nine and 12 years of age. The EEG is markedly abnormal and a low rate of intermittent photic stimulation at 1-2 flashes per second elicits characteristic, if not 'diagnostic', high-amplitude occipital spikes. The electroretinogram (ERG) is extinguished and MRI demonstrates progressive atrophy of the cerebellar and, less obviously, cerebral hemispheres. The diagnosis may be confirmed by either skin or rectal biopsy (showing the typical 'curvilinear bodies' on electron microscopy) or less invasively, by a marked deficiency of blood lysosomal tripeptidyl peptidase 1. The gene has been mapped to chromosome 15 (15q 21-23). Piracetam may be very effective in suppressing the polymyoclonia in the early stages of this condition.

Huntington's disease

The juvenile form of Huntington's disease has a different presentation to that in adults and presents between nine and 12 years of age (occasionally earlier) with seizures (myoclonic and tonic-clonic and even with episodes of convulsive status epilepticus) or cognitive impairment (Osborne, *et al.*,1982). If seizures are not prominent at presentation, the cognitive impairment and behaviour problems may lead to an initial diagnosis of a primary conduct disorder and psychiatric referral. Bradykinesia and rigidity subsequently develop and are rapidly followed by involuntary movements, ataxia and dementia. The father is affected in the vast majority of children who have the juvenile form; however, the diagnosis may not have been made or may not have been disclosed in the father when the child first presents. The genetic defect is a trinucleotide repeat (expansion) on the short arm of chromsome 4 (4p), and can be readily identified by DNA analysis.

Unverricht-Lundborg disease (also known as Baltic myoclonus)

This is one of the causes of a progressive myoclonic epilepsy presenting between the age of six and 16 years with either primary generalized tonic-clonic seizures (50% of cases) or myoclonic seizures (50% of cases). The myoclonus is often induced by action (or even the *intention* of action or movement), some sensory stimuli and or sustained posture and progresses inexorably so that the young adult is almost totally incapacitated and death usually occurs by 30-40 years of age. Some patients may also develop other seizure types, specifically absences and 'drop attacks'. Cognitive and intellectual function is initially preserved but some years after presentation cognitive deterioration may develop which is usually mild, although dementia may occur. The use of phenytoin dramatically exacerbates the myoclonus and may also contribute to any progressive cognitive impairment in these patients. Neuropathological studies reveal diffuse neuronal degeneration and Purkinje cell loss in the cerebellum but no obvious abnormal storage material. The gene has been mapped to chromosome 21q.

Lafora body disease

The clinical presentation of this progressive myoclonic epilepsy is not dissimilar to that of Unverricht-Lundborg disease. In over 75% of patients presentation is between six and 19 years of age again with epileptic seizures that are predominantly myoclonic, clonic or tonic-clonic in type but over 50% of patients will manifest partial seizures with visual symptoms. Photosensitivity is commonly found and is associated with a marked photomyoclonic response. The frequent myoclonus is also exacerbated by movement and even the intention of movement. Cognitive impairment, learning disability and dementia eventually occur but may not develop for many years after presentation – including into early adulthood. The disorder is progressive and death usually occurs within five to 10 years after onset – but generally no later than 20-25 years of age. Diagnosis is confirmed by biopsies of skin, or other tissue, that demonstrate Lafora (amyloid) bodies. These are circular, basophilic PAS (periodic acid Schiff)-positive inclusions found within neurons, liver, muscle and sweat glands of the skin. The disease is inherited as an autosomal recessive trait and the gene has been mapped to chromosome 6q 23-25.

Neurocutaneous syndromes

Most, if not all, of the neurocutaneous syndromes feature the combination of epilepsy and learning difficulties that typically are mild to severe. The epilepsy in these syndromes is usually polymorphous (many different seizure types) and is extremely difficult to control.

Most of the neurocutaneous syndromes are genetically determined (Aicardi, 1998). These commonly include:

- tuberous sclerosis (Appleton and Fryer, 1995)
- Sturge-Weber syndrome (Kramer, *et al.*, 2000)
- neurofibromatosis (Type 1)
- linear sebaceous naevus syndrome
- hypomelanosis of Ito
- incontinenta pigmenti

Miscellaneous chromosomal disorders

A large number of chromosomal disorders may be associated with both epilepsy and severe learning difficulties (Singh, *et al.*, 2002). The more common ones are listed below:

Down's syndrome (Trisomy 21): epilepsy occurs in 5-10% of patients and there is a clear association with infantile spasms affecting 1-13% of individuals (Stafstrom and Konkol, 1994). Infantile spasms account for approximately 5-50% of all seizures in people with Down's syndrome. Seizure types in older children include myoclonic, atonic, tonic-clonic and rarely, partial seizures. There does not appear to be an increased risk of early dementia (including Alzheimer's disease) in those with childhood-onset epilepsy – in contrast to adult patients with Down's syndrome who develop epilepsy after the age of 35 or 40 years of age, where there is an increased risk of early dementia (Puri and Singh, 2001).

Fragile X (Xq27.3): epilepsy occurs in 30-40% of patients, usually in early childhood on a pre-existing background of severe learning difficulties and autistic features. The dysmorphic somatic features that characterize this syndrome tend to be easier to recognize after puberty. Seizure types may be multiple but include infantile spasms, tonic-clonic and atonic.

Ring chromosome 20: a rare but probably under-diagnosed disorder that presents in mid to late childhood or adolescence with complex partial (with frontal or temporal semiology), and secondarily generalized tonic-clonic seizures, and episodes of convulsive but more frequently, non-convulsive status epilepticus (Augustijn, *et al.*, 2001). There are few dysmorphic features although most patients are microcephalic. Early development is normal but progressive cognitive difficulties often develop in those patients with an early onset of epilepsy, particularly if complicated by frequent and drug-resistant episodes of non-convulsive status epilepticus.

Ring chromosome 14: less common than ring chromosome 20 with slightly more obvious dysmorphic facial features (high, wide forehead, narrow, elongated face, microcephaly), frequent retinal dystrophy, and a high frequency of complex partial and generalized tonic-clonic seizures. Learning disability is common and is usually severe. A number of non-specific brain abnormalities have been reported including cortical atrophy, porencephaly and a dysplastic corpus callosum.

Wolf-Hirschhorn syndrome (4p 16.3 deletion): a very rare but possibly under-recognised disorder comprising of dysmorphic facial features, moderately severe or severe mental handicap, epilepsy (that may improve with age) and varying other anomalies (cardiac defects, clefts of lip and palate and sensorineural deafness) (Battaglia *et al.*, 1999).

MISCELLANEOUS SPORADIC DISORDERS

Subacute sclerosing panencephalitis (SSPE)

Although rare, this late complication of measles continues to occur with an annual incidence of approximately one per million. The decline in the incidence of SSPE is considered to be directly related to the use of measles immunization. New cases of SSPE appear to occur in those children who were infected in the first year of life before they were due to receive the immunization or in those who were not immunized and then contracted measles under two or three years of age. Males seem to be more commonly affected. Presentation may be as young as four years, but is more commonly between 10 and 16 years of age (Dyken, 2001; Garg, 2002; Ozturk, *et al.*, 2002).

The onset is often insidious, with behavioural features and a decline in school performance, but may be almost explosive, particularly in younger children. Not infrequently this may lead to an initial psychological or psychiatric referral. Subsequently children develop motor problems including clumsiness and ataxia. Seizures may be either myoclonic or tonic-clonic and become increasingly frequent; the frequent myoclonic seizures contribute to the clumsiness and ataxia. Dysphagia and dysarthria are additional early problems followed by progressive dementia, cortical visual impairment and tetraplegia leading to an almost persistent vegetative state. Death may occur from weeks to some years following presentation but 5% may spontaneously plateau and even improve; it is possible that the use of isoprinisine or beta interferon may contribute to this improvement. The diagnosis of SSPE is made on the basis of the clinical features, EEG appearance (showing characteristic periodic, high-amplitude, triphasic, sharp and slow wave complexes recurring every 3-10 seconds, particularly during hyperventilation), subtle white matter changes on MRI (particularly in the parietal and occipital regions) and definitively, by demonstrating elevated measles antibodies in the CSF.

REFERENCES

Aicardi, J. (1998). *Diseases of the Nervous System in Childhood, 2nd edn.* MacKeith Press, Cambridge.

Appleton, R.E. and Fryer, A.E. (1995). Neurological manifestations of tuberous sclerosis complex. *CNS Drugs* **3**, 174-185.

Appleton, R.E. (2001) West syndrome: long-term prognosis and social aspects. *Brain Dev* **23**, 688-691.

Augustijn, P.B., Parra, J., Wouters, C.H., Joosten, P., Lindhout, D. and Van-Emde-Boas, W. (2001). Ring chromosome 20 epilepsy syndrome in children: electroclinical features. *Neurology* **25**, 1108-1111.

Battaglia, A., Carey, J.C., Cederholm, P., Viskochil, D.H., Brothman, A.R. and Galasso, C. (1999). Natural history of Wolf-Hirschhorn syndrome: experience with 15 cases. *Pediatrics* **103**, 830-836.

Baxter, P., Griffiths, P., Kelly, T. and Gardner-Medwin, D. (1996). Pyridoxine dependent seizures: demographic, clinical, MRI and psychometric features, and effect of dose on intelligence quotient. *Dev Med Child Neurol* **38**, 998-1006.

Chiron, C., Dumas, C., Jambaque, I., Mumford, J. and Dulac, O. (1997). Randomised trial comparing vigabatrin and hydrocortisone in infantile spasms due to tuberous sclerosis. *Epil Res* **26**, 389-395.

Clark, G.D. (2001). Cerebral gyral dysplasia: molecular genetics and cell biology. *Curr Opin Neurol* **142**, 157-162.

Coppola, G., Plouin, P., Chiron, C., Robain, O. and Dulac, O. (1995). Migrating partial seizures in infancy: a malignant disorder with developmental arrest. *Epilepsia* **36**, 1017-1024.

Crino, P.B., Miyata, H. and Vintners, H.V. (2002). Neurodevelopmental disorders as a cause of seizures: neuropathological, genetic and mechanistic considerations. *Brain Path* **12**, 212-233.

Crumrine, P.K. (2002) Lennox-Gastaut syndrome. *J Child Neurol* **17** (Suppl 1), S70-S75.

Dunn, H.G. and MacLeod, P.M. (2001). Rett syndrome: review of biological abnormalities. *Can J Neurol Sci* **28**, 16-29.

Dyken, P.R. (2001). Neuroprogressive disease of post-infectious origin: a review of a resurging subacute sclerosing panencephalitis (SSPE). *Ment Retard Dev Disabil Res* **7**, 217-225.

Garg, R.K. (2002) Subacute sclerosing panencephalitis. *Postgrad Med J* **78**, 63-70.

Gropman, A.L. (2001). Diagnosis and treatment of childhood mitochondrial disease. *Curr Neurol Neurosci Rep* **1**, 185-194.

Guerrini, R. and Carrozzo, R. (2001). Epilepsy and genetic malformations of the cerebral cortex. *Am J Med Genet* **106**, 160-173.

Jan, M.M., Dooley, J.M. and Gordon, K.E. (1999). Male Rett syndrome variant: application of diagnostic criteria. *Pediatr Neurol* **20**, 238-240.

Kanazawa, O. (2001). Refractory grand mal seizures with onset during infancy including severe myoclonic epilepsy in infancy. *Brain Dev* **23**, 749-756.

Kolski, H. and Otsubo, H. (2002). The Landau-Kleffner syndrome. *Adv Exp Med Biol* **497**, 195-208.

Kramer, U., Kahana, E., Shorer, Z. and Ben-Zeer, B. (2000). Outcome of infants with unilateral Sturge-Weber syndrome and early onset seizures. *Dev Med Child Neurol* **42**, 756-759.

Laan, L.A., van-Haeringen, A. and Brouwer, O.F. (1999). Angelman syndrome: a review of clinical and genetic aspects. *Clin Neurol Neurosurg* **101**, 161-170.

Lyon, G., Adams, R.D. and Kolodny, E.H. (1996). *Neurology of Hereditary Metabolic Diseases of Children, 2nd edn.* McGraw-Hill, New York.

Niedermeyer, E. (2002). Lennox-Gastaut syndrome. Clinical description and diagnosis. *Adv Exp Med Biol* **497**, 61-75.

Osborne, J.P., Munson, P. and Burman, D. (1982). Huntington's chorea; report of 3 cases and review of the literature. *Arch Dis Child* **57**, 99-103.

Ozturk, A., Gurses, C., Baylean, B., Gokyigit, A. and Eraksoy, M. (2002). Subacute sclerosing panencephalitis: clinical and magnetic resonance imaging evaluation in 36 patients. *J Child Neurol* **17**, 25-27.

Pilz, D., Stoodley, N. and Golden, J.A. (2002). Neuronal migration, cerebral cortical development and cerebral cortical anomalies. *J Neuropath Exp Neurol* **61**, 1-11

Puri, B.K. and Singh, I. (2001). Age of seizure onset in adults with Down's syndrome. *Int J Clin Practice* **55**, 442-444.

Riikonen, R. (2001). Long-term outcome of patients with West syndrome. *Brain Dev* **23**, 683-687.

Robinson, R.O., Baird, G., Robinson, G. and Simonoff, E. (2001). Landau-Kleffner syndrome: course and correlates with outcome. *Dev Med Child Neurol* **43**, 243-247.

Roger, J., Bureau, M., Dravet, Ch., Dreifuss, F.E., Perret, A. and Wolf, P. (1992). *Epileptic Syndromes in Infancy, Childhood and Adolescence, 2nd edn.* John Libbey & Co Ltd, London.

Scheffer, I.E. and Berkovic, S.F. (1997). Generalised epilepsy with febrile seizures plus. A genetic disorder with heterogeneous clinical phenotypes. *Brain* **120**, 479-490.

Singh, R., Scheffer, I.E., Crossland, K. and Berkovic, SF. (1999). Generalised epilepsy with febrile seizures plus: a common childhood-onset genetic epilepsy syndrome. *Ann Neurol* **45**, 75-81.

Singh, R., Andermann, E., Whitehouse, W.P., Harvey, A.S., Keene, D.L., Seni, M.H., Crossland, K.M., Andermann, F., Berkovic, S.F. and Scheffer, I.E. (2001). Severe myoclonic epilepsy of infancy: extended spectrum of GEFS+? *Epilepsia* **42**, 837-844.

Singh, R., Gardner, R.J.M., Crossland, K.M., Scheffer, I.E. and Berkovic, S.F. (2002). Chromosomal abnormalities and epilepsy: a review for clinicians and gene hunters. *Epilepsia* **43**, 127-140.

Stafstrom, C.E. and Konkol, R.J. (1994). Infantile spasms in children with Down syndrome. *Dev Med Child Neurol* **36**, 576-585.

Williams, C.A., Lossie, A. and Driscoll, D. (2001). Angelman syndrome: mimicking conditions and phenotypes. *Am J Med Genet* **101**, 59-64.

West, W.J. (1841). On a peculiar form of infantile convulsions. *Lancet* **1**, 724-725.

Wong, M. and Trevathan, E. (2001). Infantile spasms. *Pediatr Neurol* **24**, 89-98.

Yamatogi, Y. and Ohtahara, S. (2002). Early infantile epileptic encephalopathy with suppression bursts, Ohtahara syndrome; its overview referring to our 16 cases. *Brain Dev* **24**, 13-23.

Learning Disability and Epilepsy: an Integrative Approach
Edited by Michael R. Trimble
© 2003 Clarius Press Ltd

5

Brain Malformations in Adults

SANJAY M. SISODIYA

Department of Clinical and Experimental Epilepsy
Institute of Neurology, University College London
Queen Square, London, UK

INTRODUCTION

The term 'malformations of cortical development' (MCD) is a contemporary description for a broad range of conditions with the common attribute of a developmental origin. Many of the component conditions have long been recognised in post-mortem studies, mainly of often grossly malformed fetuses. This led to a general belief that such malformations were rare, usually severe and often fatal. Over the last decade, the widespread availability of high quality *in vivo* neuroimaging in the form of magnetic resonance imaging (MRI) and its common use in imaging the brain in epilepsy, has led to a re-evaluation of the importance of malformations in epilepsy, learning disability and other putatively developmental brain disorders (Barkovich *et al.*, 2001). It has become clear that MCD are in fact much more common than previously appreciated, that MCD come in a broad variety of forms, and that their discovery in the individual patient may have a number of implications for management. The combination of neuroimaging with clinical and genetic studies has led to the discovery of novel genes involved in human brain development and function. This is an area of growing importance both for clinical practice and basic science (Guerrini and Carrozzo, 2002). (see Figure 1 and Table 1).

MCD is a slightly clumsy term, but its widespread usage has served to emphasise the importance of considering developmental brain anomalies in the causation of numerous conditions, and in this sense it is a useful label. With increasing detail of both investigations and understanding, more useful classification schema have been devised for the component malformations. Some classifications require pathological information about the

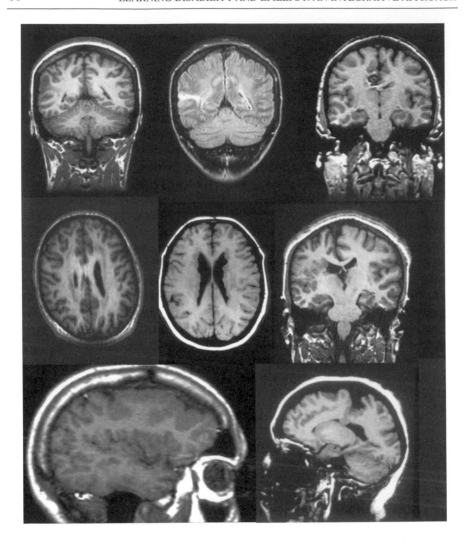

Figure 1. The figure illustrates some of the malformations discussed in the text.

Top left and middle, focal cortical dysplasia showing blurring of the grey-white interface on T1 weighted imaging and increased signal tapering down to the ventricle on FLAIR. Top right, a dysembryoplastic neuroepithelial tumour in the right cingulate gyrus.

Middle row, left, coronal image showing bilateral subcortical band hetero-topia; middle, coronal image showing bilateral periventricular nodular heterotopia; right, unilateral non-band subcortical heterotopia with overlying cortical abnormality on coronal image.

Bottom left, frontal polymicrogyria on a parasagittal image; bottom right, schizencephaly.

Table 1. Genetic basis of malformations of cortical development

Syndrome	Locus	Gene	Protein
ILS	Xq22.3-q23	*DCX = XLIS*	DCX or doublecortin
SBH	Xq22.3-q23	*DCX = XLIS*	DCX or doublecortin
MDS	17p13.3	Several contiguous	PAFAH1B1 and others
ILS	17p13.3	*LIS1*	PAFAH1B1
SBH	17p13.3	*LIS1*	PAFAH1B1
LCH	7q22	*RELN*	reelin
FCMD	9q31	*FCMD*	FCMD or fukutin
MED	1p32	Unknown	Unknown
BPNH	Xq28	*FLM1*	Falimin-1
TSC1	9q32	*TSC1*	hamartin
TSC2	16p13.3	*TSC2*	tuberin

ILS – isolated lissencephaly sequence; SBH = subcortial band heterotopi;
MDS = Miller-Dieker syndrome; LCH = lissencephaly with cerebellar hypoplasia;
FCMD – Fukyama congenital muscular dystrophy; MED = muscle-eye-brain disease,
BPNH = bilateral periventricular nodular heterotopia.

malformation to be available: in practice, it is unusual to be able to examine the malformed brain tissue under the microscope. The most useful classification is that by the doyen of imaging studies of human MCD, AJ Barkovich, and colleagues (Barkovich *et al.*, 2001). This scheme has the advantage of requiring only imaging data for its use, whilst being also flexible and informative. This chapter will consider the more common MCD in the framework provided by this classification.

The Barkovich classification attempts to order MCD according to fundamental biological processes into three major groups: those resulting from abnormalities of cell proliferation, those resulting from abnormalities of neuronal migration, and those resulting from abnormal cortical organisation.

Only with further research will it become clear if the categories chosen are all correct. However, the classification makes it clear that MCD cannot be alternatively grouped under the blanket term 'neuronal migration disorders', as not all are due to anomalies of migration; nor is it appropriate to call them 'cortical dysplasia' as has been commonly the case: both are erroneous loose misnomers and should now be avoided. It is important also to remember that in some cases, classification proves impossible, and that histologically more than one MCD may be seen in the same tissue – for example heterotopia and polymicrogyria. The resulting clinical phenotype may be difficult to predict.

Given that as far as current understanding allows, MCD result from disruption of the processes of proliferation, migration and organisation, it is not surprising that such conditions should manifest with alteration in brain function – specifically in epilepsy, learning disability or motor disorders. One series suggests MCD may be seen in 14% of individuals with epilepsy and learning disability (Brodtkorb *et al.*, 1992).

It is perhaps surprising that MCD are not more commonly the cause of a broader range of problems. In fact, it is likely that MCD, possibly of varieties not yet commonly recognised (eg synaptic malformation), and not yet identifiable on imaging (eg microdysgenesis) or those sometimes missed currently even on detailed high-resolution MRI (eg subtle focal cortical dysplasia), are the cause of localisation-related epilepsy or learning disorders that are currently considered cryptogenic (Sisodiya, 2000). Thus MCD are likely to prove of greater significance as both *in vivo* imaging and basic understanding advance and it is of value for physicians caring for people with epilepsy, learning disability, or both, to have a general knowledge of MCD. The basic premise implicit in consideration of learning disability associated with MCD is that the disruption of the normal structure and function of the brain in MCD causing epilepsy also underlies the learning disability. The links may be more subtle, and certainly in childhood, developmental arrest or regression may occur partly as a result of frequent clinical or subclinical seizures as part of an epileptic encephalopathy. This phenomenon would seem to be very rare, if it occurs at all, in adulthood.

In the discussions that follow, learning disability will be considered to be that present in association with the MCD, rather than any acquired difficulties arising from the consequences of epilepsy (eg acquired hippocampal damage), secondary head injury or the effects of antiepileptic drugs on cognition or metabolism (eg hyperammonaemic encephalopathy secondary to valproate treatment). Nevertheless, these confounding issues always need to be borne in mind in clinical practice when addressing the problems that may present.

CLASSIFICATION SCHEME FOR MCD

There are many malformations classified in the scheme of Barkovich *et al.* (2001)   (Table 2). Only some are considered below: these are seen most commonly in epilepsy practice. Some are subclassified in the original scheme, to which the interested reader is referred: for most of these subdivisions, there is relatively little additional information available.

Table 2. Classification scheme

I. Malformation due to abnormal neuronal and glial proliferation or apoptosis

   A. Decreased Proliferation/Increased Apoptosis: Microcephalises

      1. Microcephaly with normal to thin cortex

      2. Microlissencephaly (extreme microcephaly with thick cortex)

   B. Increased Proliferation/Decreased Apoptosis (normal cell types): Megalencephalies

   C. Abnormal Proliferation (abnormal cell types)

      1. Non-neoplastic

         a. Cortical hamartomas of tuberous sclerosis

         b. Cortical dysplasia with balloon cells

         c. Hemimegalencephaly (HMEG)

      2. Neoplastic (associated with disordered cortex)

         a. DNET (dysembryoplastic neuroepithelial tumor)

         b. Ganglioglioma

         c. Gangliocytoma

II. Malformation due to abnormal neuronal migration

   A. Lissencephaly/Subcortical Band Heterotopia Spectrum

   B. Cobblestone complex

      1. Congenital muscular dystrophy syndromes

      2. Syndromes with no involvement of muscle

   C. Heterotopia

      1. Subependymal (periventricular)

      2. Subcortical (other than Band Heterotopia)

      3. Marginal glioneuronal

continued

Table 2.   continued from previous page.

III. Malformations due to abnormal cortical organisation (including later neuronal migration)

    A. Polymicrogyria and schizencephaly

        1. Bilateral polymicrogyria syndromes

        2. Schizencephaly (polymicrogyria with clefts)

        3. Polymicrogyria with other brain malformations or abnormalities

        4. Polymicrogyria or schizencephaly as part of Multiple Congenital Anomaly/Mental Retardation syndromes

    B. Cortical dysplasia without balloon cells

    C. Microdysgenesis

IV. Malformations of cortical development, not otherwise classified

    A. Malformations secondary to inborn errors of metabolism

        1. Mitochondrial and pyruvate metabolic disorders

        2. Peroxisomal disorders

    B. Other unclassified malformations

        1. Sublobar dysplasia

        2. Others

IC1a: Tuberous Sclerosis

This condition is not considered in this chapter, as it has long been recognised to be associated with epilepsy and learning disability. The reader is referred to excellent monographs and recent research articles for further information (see www.tuberous-sclerosis.org).

IC1b: Focal cortical dysplasia; IIIB: focal cortical dysplasia without balloon cell glia

Focal cortical dysplasia (FCD) was first reported by Taylor and colleagues in 1971 (Taylor *et al.*, 1971). It has since become clear that it is one of the most common MCD found either on imaging studies in patients with refractory epilepsy, or in surgical resection specimens, even accounting for the inherent bias in surgical series. As originally described, before the advent of modern neuroimaging, FCD consisted of an area or areas of disordered cortical lamina-tion, blurring of the grey-white matter boundary, the presence of malorientated, misplaced pyramidal neurons and giant, dysplastic neurons, as well as balloon cell glia with indistinct cell boundaries and a glassy cytoplasm. This morphological characterisation has changed little since.

More recently, FCD has been the focus of a range of imaging, neuropathological and molecular genetic studies addressing its aetiology and pathophysiology (Tassi et al., 2002). As with all conditions of essentially unknown aetiology, lumping and splitting have occurred. Barkovich and colleagues' classification divides FCD into two groups, one in which the characteristic balloon cell glia are present pathologically (grouped under MCD with abnormalities of proliferation) and one in which they are absent (grouped under MCD with abnormalities of organisation). This may eventually turn out to be justifiable, and indeed there are additional pathological, imaging and clinical data to suggest these varieties may differ. For the purposes of discussion of FCD in relation to learning disability, the two types are considered together here, as in practical terms the presence or absence of balloon cell glia appears to have little impact on prognosis or surgical outcome to date, though some more recent publications suggest this may not be the case, for example Tassi et al. (2002).

In contrast to most other MCD, FCD is invariably associated with epilepsy, and such epilepsy is often refractory to treatment. This is not simply a referral bias: many thousands of normal individuals have had MRI brain scans in various studies and trials, and to the author's knowledge, no asymptomatic cases of FCD have been reported in the English language literature. It must be assumed therefore that FCD is potently epileptogenic. Intrinsic epileptogenicity has been shown for FCD in a number of studies (for a review, see Sisodiya, 2000).

MRI studies can identify FCD in many, but not all, cases. The gold standard for its detection remains histopathology, in cases where this is available. Experience shows that FCD may be associated with varying degrees of learning disability. Reviews and larger series suggest that perhaps a third of cases have learning disability, but many series consist of selected cases, for example operable cases only. Thus the true incidence of learning disability associated with FCD is unknown, not least because the true prevalence of FCD is also unknown.

The basis of the epileptogenicity of FCD is unknown. The extent of FCD in a given individual is also often unknown. Though the qualifier 'focal' is part of the name of this MCD, in fact Taylor and colleagues (Taylor et al., 1971) in their original report recognised that in some cases it was multifocal even within a temporal lobectomy specimen, and that further noncontiguous foci could not be discounted: it may well be that other, if less ostentatious, areas of cortical dysplasia could have been left behind after focal resection. This possibility is supported by the fact that even within the limits of the resected lobes the abnormality was sometimes disseminated rather than confined to a single patch. The degree, therefore, to which the brain as a whole may be affected remains uncertain.

Indeed, this propensity has been blamed for the comparatively poor outcome after therapeutic focal resection of FCD (Sisodiya, 2000). Many (at least 25%) cases of FCD are not seen on MRI. By extrapolation, it is likely that the entire extent of FCD is not apparent when a single abnormal area is visualised on MRI: this has been demonstrated pathologically.

This widespread extent of FCD may explain the association with learning disability. Most surgical series do not allow determination of whether associated learning disability is an adverse prognostic factor for surgical outcome, but these considerations would suggest that it is. Some of the many reported intriguing molecular derangements in FCD may underlie the learning disability seen, through more widespread neuronal and network dysfunction.

FCD presenting in infancy may behave differently and be responsible for catastrophic refractory epilepsy associated with developmental regression. In such cases, epilepsy surgery may be life-saving as well as curative, and many authorities would recommend early intervention in this situation. The normal maturation of white matter in early life can obscure FCD, initially highlighted by its intrinsic signal abnormalities set amongst the surrounding unmyelinated infant brain tissue, and careful review of MRI is necessary in infants with refractory localisation-related epilepsy. Positron emission tomography or SPECT may also be of some localising value in this situation (Chugani, 1992; Cross et al., 1997).

Histopathologically, FCD may be indistinguishable from tuberous sclerosis. This has led to an examination of single nucleotide polymorphisms in the genes causing tuberous sclerosis (hamartin and tuberin) in pooled single dysplastic FCD neurons, with some suggestion that changes in these genes may also explain dysplasia in FCD (Becker et al., 2002). Conversely, it may be perhaps that learning disability in tuberous sclerosis is due to invisible widespread malformation beyond the obvious cortical tubers alone.

IC1c: Hemimegalencephaly

Debate continues about the nosology of hemimegalencephaly (Flores-Sarnat, 2002). It may occur in association with a variety of other congenital anomalies, including linear sebaceous nevus, hypomelanosis of Ito and hemihypertrophy syndromes and tuberous sclerosis. Histologically, the underlying malformation can usually be classified under one of the other categories. It is likely that the epileptogenesis depends on the underlying malformation, which is closest in most cases to focal cortical dysplasia, though abnormalities are obviously more widespread. Indeed in at least one case, malformation was also was found at postmortem in an apparently normal contralateral hemisphere (Jahan et al., 1997).

Learning disability is common in hemimegalencephaly. This may reflect grossly (and bilaterally) disordered cerebral development. It may also be that frequent epileptic activity spreading to the otherwise apparently normal hemisphere limits the functional maturation of that hemisphere. Thus, after hemispherectomy, there may be developmental catch-up. In one dramatic case, late acquisition of language was documented after surgery (Vargha-Khadem *et al.*, 1997). It is interesting to speculate whether this phenomenon may be occurring with other brain malformations, but it is rarely feasible to test this hypothesis by surgical intervention in malformations other than hemimegalencephaly or cortical dysplasia with onset of epilepsy in infancy.

Accordingly, surgical treatment is usually by functional hemispherectomy. This is usually only contemplated in the presence of hemiparesis. Though the contralateral hemisphere usually appears normal, the presence of independent epileptiform changes over it preoperatively is held by some to suggest the presence of additional pathology, manifest by a poorer outcome (Smith *et al.*, 1991), though others do not find this (Döring *et al.*, 1999).

IC2a: Dysembryoplastic neuroepithelial tumours

Dysembryoplastic neuroepithelial tumours (DNTs) are cortically-based lesions, with specific histological and radiological features, responsible for refractory epilepsy, and considered a "neoplastic derivative from cortical matrix" rather than a hamartoma. Marked by benignity, surgery offers effective epilepsy treatment, adjunctive chemotherapy or radiotherapy being unnecessary (Daumas-Duport *et al.*, 1988). Some 200 cases generally conforming to this stereotype have been published. The diagnostic spectrum has been widened, recent criteria emphasising clinical rather than histological aspects (Daumas-Duport *et al.*, 1999). Many cases, however, remain unreported, because recognition is simple and treatment effective.

DNTs usually cause localisation-related epilepsy before the age of 20. Neurological signs are absent, or minor and stable (Raymond *et al.*, 1995). The epilepsy is almost always refractory to drug treatment, notwithstanding reporting bias. There are characteristic findings on neuroimaging, with a lesion often of mixed signal characteristics on MRI, based in cortex, possibly involving white matter, often with overlying skull changes suggesting the lesion has been present for many years (Daumas-Duport *et al.*, 1999). DNTs may be associated with other epileptogenic abnormalities, such as hippocampal sclerosis, and rarely may be extensive and complex, extending beyond the usual location in frontal or temporal lobes.

Findings with respect to epileptogenesis are variable. Surgical treatment very commonly renders patients seizure-free (140/167 cases seizure-free at one year; 53/60 cases free at two years; literature reviewed to January 2000), suggesting the DNT is necessary for epileptogenesis. However, EEG, electrocorticographic and magnetoencephalographic findings are often contradictory. These are incomplete and unexplained findings. Remarkably, the extent of resection of the DNT and the presence of additional pathologies appears not to influence outcome, in stark contrast to outcome for other malformations treated surgically (Honavar *et al.*, 1999). The reason for this intriguing finding is unknown.

The characteristic histopathological features of DNT include a predominant intracortical location with a classically multinodular architecture, although diffuse forms of DNT have been recently reported (Honavar *et al.*, 1999). The cellular composition of these tumours is mixed, including glial cells, oligodendrocyte-like cells (OLCs) and neurones located both within nodules and in a separate and pathognomonic 'glioneuronal element'. Despite a rather complex and heterogenous appearance within any individual tumour, consistent and quite uniform patterns are recognised between cases. A more variable finding in DNT studies has been the identification of dysplasia in the adjacent resected cortex (Honavar *et al.*, 1999). Dysplasia and the quasi-hamartomatous appearance of these glio-neuronal tumours has led to the assumption that they arise on the background of a malformed cortex. The descriptions of the malformation adjacent to DNT includes microdysgenesis, glioneuronal hamartias (or microdysgenetic nodules), and occasionally grey matter heterotopias and cortical dysplasia with giant neurons.

Published imaging and pathological features leave the origin of DNTs obscure. They are probably developmental, being found as early as two weeks of life. There is often thinning or indenting of the calvarium, and associated reorganized cortical function. The coexistence of FCD, neuronal heterotopia, microdysgenesis and neurofibromatosis supports a developmental origin.

Learning disability may be part of the clinical presentation (15% of cases; Degen *et al.*, 2002). The implications for the complex biology of DNTs are not clear. However, in terms of management, it is clear that the presence of learning disability, suggesting as usual widespread cortical dysfunction, is a contraindication to surgical resection of any or part of the DNT. The outcome in such cases is uniformly poor both in terms of control of the epilepsy and behaviour. This is in contrast to the existence of learning disability or developmental regression in some other malformations, which in fact may encourage consideration of surgery.

IIA: Lissencephaly/subcortical band heterotopia spectrum

Lissencephaly describes a smooth brain without gyration (agyria), or with decreased gyration (pachygyria): it may affect part of the brain, anteriorly or posteriorly predominant, or all of it. The cortex is thickened. There may be difficultly in distinguishing lissencephaly from polymicrogyria, or other rarer abnormalities, on neuroimaging in inexperienced hands. Subcortical band heterotopia is marked by a gyral pattern that is usually simplified, beneath which a thin band of white matter separates an inner kernel of neurons arrested in migration and forming a band of variable convolutedness, thickness and extent.

On first analysis, these conditions might be considered morphologically quite distinct. MRI, however, has shown this is incorrect. Imaging of kindreds with males affected by often devastating epilepsy and marked learning disability and affected females with a less severe phenotype has shown that in some such kindreds females have subcortical band (or laminar) heterotopia, fancifully designated 'the double cortex syndrome', whilst the more severely affected males have lissencephaly (Barkovich *et al.*, 2001). The pattern suggests an X-linked inheritance with a more severe phenotype in males, and traditional linkage studies have identified mutations in most of these kindreds of a completely novel gene influencing brain development, known as doublecortin (*DCX*) (Gleeson, 2001).

Lissencephaly is a severe developmental abnormality, that may form part of a syndrome, the most common of which is the Miller-Dieker syndrome. The neurological phenotype in classical lissencephaly is severe: patients rarely survive beyond the first two decades. Learning disability and developmental delay are usually profound; there may be spastic quadraparesis; 90% of affected children have epilepsy. Such epilepsy usually manifests with infantile spasms, and subsequently a mixture of seizure types develops, possibly with persisting spasms. The EEG may be characteristic, featuring fast rhythms of particularly high amplitude.

In subcortical band heterotopia, patients usually have epilepsy and learning disability. The severity of the latter relates to the extent and thickness of the subcortical band (Barkovich and Kjos, 1992). The majority of patients (90%) have seizures, with a variety of seizure types. Often the epilepsy is refractory to drug treatment.

MRI usually clearly delineates the nature and extent of the malformation. Detailed examination of the malformation is important as, in concert with clinical and EEG findings, MRI will shape the investigational strategy (Guerrini and Carrozzo, 2002). When subcortical band heterotopia occurs in X-linked dominant fashion, with greater severity or lissencephaly in affected males, mutations in *DCX* (an X-linked gene) are likely, having been reported in all such kindreds studied. DCX mutations account also for 40-90% of sporadically affected female patients with subcortical band heterotopia. The band heterotopia or pachygyria is more predominant anteriorly on MRI in these cases. Rarely, band heterotopia in males may be due to *DCX* mutations. For patients with classical isolated lissencephaly (isolated lissencephaly sequence, ILS), mutations in another novel gene, *LIS1* (chromosome 17), are found in 65% of patients. The malformation (pachygyria, agyria) is more predominant posteriorly on MRI in subjects with *LIS1* mutation.

Investigation of patients with these malformations should be undertaken at a specialist center, and may include chromosome analysis, fluorescent *in situ* hybridization and direct gene sequencing. These will be informed by pedigree analysis and consideration of syndromic diagnoses. Counselling will be required: mothers or female relatives of patients with *DCX* mutation may have an occult heritable mutation in the presence of an apparently normal MRI brain scan.

IIC1: Periventricular nodular heterotopia (PVNH)

Though recognised for over a century, it is again due to the widespread use of MRI that the prevalence of PVNH has become appreciated. PVNH is also known as subependymal heterotopia, describing collections of neurons grouped together to form masses immediately underlying or close to the ependyma of the lateral ventricles (Raymond *et al.*, 1994). The masses may appear as distinct nodules or more coalesced bumpy band-like structures; they may be single or multiple, symmetric or not, and may be associated with other malformations, including hippocampal abnormalities, subcortical nodules and overlying cortical changes. Seizures may originate from the nodules or the overlying grey matter, which are probably connected. The nodules can be distinguished from other lesions found at the same location by the fact that on all sequences the nodules have the same signal intensity as grey matter. Accurate differential diagnosis is important for patient counselling: misdiagnosing PVNH as tuberous sclerosis can have important consequences.

The use of MRI as a phenotyping tool, as in studies of lissencephaly and band heterotopia, has allowed traditional linkage studies to be undertaking in families in which epilepsy and PVNH co-segregate. In turn, this led to the identification of filamin A (*FLNA*) as the gene mutation which causes X-linked familial PVNH (Fox *et al.*, 1998). This condition features relatively symmetrical nodular PVNH underlying the lateral ventricles, especially in the trigones of the lateral ventricles, and is characterised clinically by the occurrence of seizures with onset in the second decade, or even later. Less commonly, cardiac anomalies and coagulopathy may be associated with this type of PVNH. X-inactivation is considered the explanation for the occurrence of PVNH in affected females, whilst the lack of a normal gene has been blamed for early fetal or neonatal lethality in affected males. Typically in PVNH associated with *FLNA* mutations, affected females are of normal intellect.

However, it has become clear that whilst most X-linked familial PVNH cases are caused by *FLNA* mutations, sporadic cases are not usually due to detectable mutations in this gene (Sheen *et al.*, 2001). In addition, there are rare familial female cases with learning disability (Musumeci *et al.*, 1997), and rare surviving males from PVNH kindreds. Genetic heterogeneity is therefore likely, and this may explain the occurrence of learning disability in some PVNH cases, particularly when the heterotopia are less nodular and more confluent. In some pedigrees, a recessive mode of inheritance is suggested. The recurrence risk in isolated cases with no demonstrated *FLNA* mutation and no imaging evidence of familial occurrence appears to be low.

PVNH has also been described in association with a variety of other syndromes, including Ehlers-Danlos syndrome, frontal-nasal dysplasia and short-gut syndrome, further supporting genetic heterogeneity in its aetiology (Guerrini and Dobyns, 1998).

The rarity of learning disability in PVNH without other brain malformation mandates exclusion of other causes of cognitive impairment, though there should rarely be any diagnostic difficulty if a good clinical history is obtained: acquired cognitive impairment has characteristics that are quite different to those of learning disability. Recognition of PVNH in a patient with learning disability, conversely, is important as imaging of relatives and genetic testing may be necessary, with appropriate counselling before and after testing.

IIC2 Non band heterotopic subcortical heterotopia

This is a comparatively rare malformation, and consequently less well studied (Barkovich, 1996). The heterotopia are nodular, but often irregular. The nodules may be single and unilateral, and perhaps quite subtle, or large, confluent, extending from cortical surface to ventricular margin, bilateral and possibly associated with additional malformations such as overlying polymicrogyria or subjacent periventricular heterotopia. The clinical manifestations differ accordingly, and the degree of learning disability is very variable. Indeed, this type of malformation illustrates how severe cerebral structural disruption and clinical phenotype are often discordant: it is not as easy to predict function from structure in this malformation as in subcortical band heterotopia. The overlying cortex may also be abnormally thin. Epilepsy may arise initially from a nodule or overlying cortex, an animal model suggests that the latter is the more important.

The abnormality is usually sporadic, and no genetic aetiology has been identified. Surgical resection has been considered, but is usually unsuccessful, which is perhaps not unsurprising given the animal data (Sisodiya, 2000). There is little guidance for generic management strategy in this MCD, and, as for many cases of MCD, individual strategies are likely to be necessary.

IIIA1 Bilateral polymicrogyria

In this condition there are, polymicrogyria is the presence of an excessive number of small gyri. The cortex on MRI may appear thickened, but the surface is usually not smooth, with irregular convolutions, usually allowing distinction from lissencephaly. It may be found in various patterns of extent and distribution, from global, through hemispheric to bilateral symmetric or more limited apparently unilateral forms (Guerrini and Carrozzo, 2002). Not surprisingly, therefore, the clinical manifestations vary and include severe learning disability, an opercular syndrome, and spastic quadraparesis, but the phenotype may also be much milder or even asymptomatic.

A variety of syndromes have been described, of which the bilateral symmetric distributions are perhaps best documented (Barkovich *et al.*, 1999). These include bilateral perisylvian polymicrogyria, bilateral frontal polymicrogyria and bilateral parasagittal parieto-occipital polymicrogyria.

Most cases are sporadic, but polymicrogyria also occurs in a number of syndromes with probable genetic aetiology, and may also be a feature of the cerebral phenotype in some rare monogenic disorders. It may occur as a result of an environmental insult, including intrauterine infection and ischaemia, or carbon monoxide poisoning .

Bilateral perisylvian polymicrogyria is associated with a characteristic MRI appearance (Kuzniecky *et al.*, 1994). It causes an opercular syndrome with faciopharyngoglossomasticatory diparesis, causing early and persistent feeding difficulties with drooling and spastic quadraparesis with marked learning difficulties in most cases. It is very probably the same condition as Worster-Drought syndrome (Clark *et al.*, 2000). The patients usually have atypical absences, tonic or atonic attacks causing drops and generalised tonic-clonic seizures. Its occurrence may be familial, though the varied patterns of inheritance suggest genetic heterogeneity. There may in some cases be an association with chromosomal abnormalities. The specific additional difficulties caused by perisylvian disease necessitate consideration of speech and language therapy for communication aids, and in some cases provision of a special diet and measures to reduce drooling (such as botulinum toxin injections).

Many other types of polymicrogyria, largely based on MRI appearances, have been described in small case series. Little is added to our knowledge of polymicrogyria by these phenotypes, and none have yet contributed to understanding of the development or treatment of epilepsy associated with polymicrogyria. In the classification scheme used to arrange this chapter, such types are grouped in 'IIIA3 polymicrogyria +' and 'IIIA4 polymicrogyria as part of multiple congenital anomaly/MR syndromes'. These are not considered further here.

IIIA2 Schizencephaly

This term means 'cleft brain', with the appearance on MRI and, if gross enough, on X-ray CT scanning, of a cleft that may extend through the entire thickness of the cortex. Clefts may be bilateral (and symmetrical or not), are usually within the central regions, and may occasionally be so subtle as to only be detected on careful analysis of high resolution imaging or, indeed, on neuropathological examination alone. The lips of the cleft(s) may be separated (open-lipped schizencephaly) or apposed (closed-lip schizencephaly). The lips forming the banks of the cleft usually contain polymicrogyric cortex, suggesting an aetiological link between the two.

Whilst the majority (80%) of patients have epilepsy, the manifestations of schizencephaly vary to some extent with the severity of the malformation. Bilateral clefts and those that are open-lipped are more likely to be associated with severe phenotypes, including microcephaly, severe developmental delay and quadraparesis, whilst more occult unilateral clefts may be asymptomatic. No particular seizure type predominates in the associated epilepsy in these subjects.

A small proportion of patients with schizencephaly were found to have *de novo* truncation or missense mutations in a developmental gene, *EMX2* (Brunelli *et al.*, 1996). However, this finding has not been replicated by other groups. In addition, clastic events *in utero*, some resulting from certain infections, may also cause schizencephaly in animal models. No definitive statements can be made about genetic counselling currently.

IIIC Microdysgenesis

This malformation cannot be identified on any current form of neuroimaging. In fact, dispute remains about its very definition. A range of subtle alterations in cortical microanatomy was described in cases of idiopathic generalised epilepsy studied at postmortem (Meencke and Veith, 1999). Subsequently, similar changes were identified in resection specimens from patients with a variety of refractory localisation-related epilepsies. Variation in definition and analysis have led to uncertainty about this malformation. Most studies use arbitrary biassed methods of quantitative analysis, or only subjective qualitative analysis. In addition, some features of microdysgenesis may be found in normal brains, to some extent: thus in normal white matter, neurons may be found, but in microdysgenesis it is claimed that there are excessive numbers of such neurons. A recent study has used stereological quantitation to more rigorously address this and similar difficulties (Thom *et al.*, 2001). It seems likely that this is indeed a real abnormality, though its provenance is unclear. If further study reveals it to have a developmental basis, microdysgenesis will be a good candidate malformation for perhaps many cases of currently cryptogenic learning disability in epilepsy.

CONCLUSIONS

Overall malformations of cortical development are not uncommon causes of epilepsy, particularly refractory epilepsy. As they may affect large areas of cortex, and cause severe electrophysiological disruption, it is also not uncommonly the case that the malformations are associated with learning disability. In fact, it is perhaps more difficult to understand why so many cases of learning disability and epilepsy in adults are not associated with apparent malformation. Subtle alterations in cortical anatomy, biochemistry and connectivity, perhaps beyond the resolution of current neuroimaging, may explain this discrepancy.

In most cases, no particular malformation is associated with a given epilepsy syndrome in the context of learning disability. Associated clinical, familial and examination findings may hint at an underlying malformation, but in most cases, the malformation is only revealed by adequately detailed neuroimaging reviewed by an experienced neuroradiologist. It has been shown that specialist imaging in an epilepsy centre changes the neuroimaging diagnosis in refractory epilepsy in a fifth of cases.

Making a specific diagnosis of a particular malformation in the context of learning disability only rarely leads to a specific treatment strategy. For the epilepsy itself, antiepileptic drug treatment remains the mainstay of treatment. The philosophy of drug use in this context is considered elsewhere in this book. In most, though not all, cases the identification of a specific malformation will not lead to novel treatment options. Surgery is usually not considered an appropriate option because the very existence of associated learning disability usually suggests more extensive derangement than can be seen on neuroimaging alone and is thus usually considered to be a marker of a poor outcome, and further because issues of consent are not insignificant. This approach, however, does not apply to epilepsy caused by certain malformations in paediatric practice, as discussed above.

However, the identification of a specific malformation is important in prognostication, explanation to the patient and relatives of the cause of the epilepsy and learning disability, and for counselling of the patient and other family members. This has become particularly important with the knowledge of underlying genetic defects and their consequences. Usually, the malformation leads to a phenotype with reproductive disadvantage, so that issues of heritability may not be of direct importance to the proband, but of potentially huge significance for other family members who may be carriers of the underlying genetic mutation.

Further study in this area may help understanding of the basis of apparently cryptogenic learning disability in epilepsy.

REFERENCES

Barkovich, A.J. (2002). Magnetic resonance imaging: role in the understanding of cerebral malformations. *Brain Dev* **24**, 2-12.

Barkovich, A.J. and Kjos, B.O. (1992). Gray matter heterotopias: MR characteristics and correlation with developmental and neurologic manifestations. *Radiology* **182**, 493-499.

Barkovich, A.J. (1996). Subcortical heterotopia: a distinct clinicoradiologic entity. *Am J Neuroradiol* **17**, 1315-1322.

Barkovich, A.J., Hevner, R. and Guerrini, R. (1999). Syndromes of bilateral symmetrical polymicrogyria. *Am J Neuroradiol* **20**, 1814-1821.

Barkovich, A.J. and Kuziecky, R.I. (2000). Gray matter heterotopia. *Neurology* **55**, 1603-1608.

Barkovich, A.J., Kuzniecky, R.I., Jackson, G.D., Guerrini, R. and Dobyns, W.B. (2001). Classification system for malformations of cortical development: update 2001. *Neurology* **57**, 2168-2178.

Becker, A.J., Urbach, H., Scheffler, B., Baden, T., Normann, S., Lahl, R., Pannek, H.W., Tuxhorn, I., Elger, C.E., Schramm, J., Wiestler, O.D. and Blumcke, I. (2002). Focal cortical dysplasia of Taylor's balloon cell type: mutational analysis of the TSC1 gene indicates a pathogenic relationship to tuberous sclerosis. *Ann Neurol* **52**, 29-37.

Brodtkorb, E., Nilsen, G., Smevik, O. and Rinck, P.A. (1992). Epilepsy and anomalies of neuronal migration: MRI and clinical aspects. *Acta Neurol Scand* **86**, 24-32.

Brunelli, S., Faiella, A., Capra, V., Nigro, V., Simeone, A., Cama, A. and Boncinelli, E. (1996). Germline mutations in the homeobox gene EMX2 in patients with severe schizencephaly. *Nat Genet* **12**, 94-96.

Chugani, H.T. (1992). The use of positron emission tomography in the clinical assessment of epilepsy. *Semin Nucl Med* **22**, 247-253.

Clark, M., Carr, L., Reilly, S. and Neville, B.G. (2000). Worster-Drought syndrome, a mild tetraplegic perisylvian cerebral palsy: review of 47 cases [In Process Citation]. *Brain* **123**, 2160-2170.

Cross, J.H., Boyd, S.G., Gordon, I., Harper, A. and Neville, B.G. (1997). Ictal cerebral perfusion related to EEG in drug resistant focal epilepsy of childhood. *J Neurol Neurosurg Psychiatry* **62**, 377-384.

Daumas-Duport, C., Scheithauer, B.W., Chodkiewicz, J.P., Laws, E.R., Jr. and Vedrenne, C. (1988). Dysembryoplastic neuroepithelial tumor: a surgically curable tumor of young patients with intractable partial seizures. Report of thirty-nine cases. *Neurosurgery* **23**, 545-556.

Daumas-Duport, C., Varlet, P., Bacha, S., Beuvon, F., Cervera-Pierot, P. and Chodkiewicz, J.P. (1999). Dysembryoplastic neuroepithelial tumors: nonspecific histological forms -- a study of 40 cases. *J Neurooncol* **41**, 267-280.

Degen, R., Ebner, A., Lahl, R., Leonhardt, S., Pannek, H.W. and Tuxhorn, I. (2002). Various findings in surgically treated epilepsy patients with dysembryoplastic neuroepithelial tumors in comparison with those of patients with other low-grade brain tumors and other neuronal migration disorders. *Epilepsia* **43**, 1379-1384.

Döring, S., Cross, H., Boyd, S., Harkness, W. and Neville, B. (1999). The significance of bilateral EEG abnormalities before and after hemispherectomy in children with unilateral major hemisphere lesions. *Epil Res* **34**, 65-73.

Flores-Sarnat, L. (2002). Hemimegalencephaly: part 1. Genetic, clinical, and imaging aspects. *J Child Neurol* **17**, 373-384.

Fox, J.W., Lamperti, E.D., Eksioglu, Y.Z., Hong, S.E., Feng, Y., Graham, D.A., Scheffer, I.E., Dobyns, W.B., Hirsch, B.A., Radtke, R.A., Berkovic, S.F., Huttenlocher, P.R. and Walsh, C.A. (1998). Mutations in filamin 1 prevent migration of cerebral cortical neurons in human periventricular heterotopia. *Neuron* **21**, 1315-1325.

Gleeson, J.G. (2001). Neuronal migration disorders. *Ment Retard Dev Disabil Res Rev* **7**(3), 167-171.

Guerrini, R. and Carrozzo, R. (2002). Epileptogenic brain malformations: clinical presentation, malformative patterns and indications for genetic testing. *Seizure* **11** *(Suppl A)*, 532-543.

Guerrini, R. and Dobyns, W.B. (1998).Bilateral periventricular nodular heterotopia with mental retardation and frontonasal malformation. *Neurology* **51**, 499-503.

Honavar, M., Janota, I. and Polkey, C.E. (1999). Histological heterogeneity of dysembryoplastic neuroepithelial tumour: identification and differential diagnosis in a series of 74 cases. *Histopathology* **34**, 342-356.

Jahan, R., Mischel, P.S., Curran, J.G., Peacock, W.J., Shields, D.W. and Vinters, H.V. (1997). Bilateral neuropathologic changes in a child with hemimegalencephaly. *Pediatr Neurol* **17**, 344-349.

Kuzniecky, R., Andermann, F. and Guerrini, R. (1994). The epileptic spectrum in the congenital bilateral perisylvian syndrome. CBPS Multicenter Collaborative Study. *Neurology* **44**, 379-385.

Meencke, H.J. and Veith, G. (1999). The relevance of slight migrational disturbances (microdysgenesis) to the etiology of the epilepsies. *Adv Neurol* **79**, 123-131.

Musumeci, S.A., Ferri, R., Elia, M., Scuderi, C., Del Gracco, S., Azan, G. and Stefanini, M.C. (1997). A new family with periventricular nodular heterotopia and peculiar dysmorphic features. A probable X-linked dominant trait. *Arch Neurol* **54**, 61-64.

Raymond, A.A., Fish, D.R., Sisodiya, S.M., Alsanjari, N., Stevens, J.M. and Shorvon, S.D. (1995). Abnormalities of gyration, heterotopias, tuberous sclerosis, focal cortical dysplasia, microdysgenesis, dysembryoplastic neuroepithelial tumour and dysgenesis of the archicortex in epilepsy. Clinical, EEG and neuroimaging features in 100 adult patients. *Brain* **118**, 629-660.

Raymond, A.A., Fish, D.R., Stevens, J.M., Sisodiya, S.M., Alsanjari, N. and Shorvon, S.D. (1994). Subependymal heterotopia: a distinct neuronal migration disorder associated with epilepsy. J Neurol Neurosurg Psychiatry **57**, 1195-1202.

Sheen, V.L., Dixon, P.H., Fox, J.W., Hong, S.E., Kinton, L., Sisodiya, S.M., Duncan, J.S., Dubeau, F. et al. (2001). Mutations in the X-linked filamin 1 gene cause periventricular nodular heterotopia in males as well as in females. *Hum Mol Genet* **10**, 1775-1783.

Sisodiya, S.M. (2000). Surgery for malformations of cortical development causing epilepsy. *Brain* **123**, 1075-1091.

Smith, S.J.M., Andermann, F., Villemure, J-G., Rasmussen, T.B. and Quesney, L.P. (1991). Functional hemispherectomy: EEG findings, spiking from isolated brain postoperatively, and prediction of outcome. *Neurology* **41**, 1790-1794.

Tassi, L., Colombo, N., Garbelli, R., Francione, S., Lo, R.G., Mai, R., Cardinale, F., Cossu, M., Ferrario, A., Galli, C., Bramerio, M., Citterio, A. and Spreafico, R. (2002). Focal cortical dysplasia: neuropathological subtypes, EEG, neuroimaging and surgical outcome. *Brain* **125**, 1719-1732.

Taylor, D.C., Falconer, M.A., Bruton, C.J. and Corsellis, J.A. (1971). Focal dysplasia of the cerebral cortex in epilepsy. *J Neurol Neurosurg Psychiatry* **34**, 369-387.

Thom, M., Sisodiya, S., Harkness, W. and Scaravilli, F. (2001). Microdysgenesis in temporal lobe epilepsy: A quantitative and immunohistochemical study of white matter neurones. *Brain* **124**, 2299-2309.

Vargha-Khadem, F., Carr, L.J., Isaacs, E., Brett, E., Adams, C. and Mishkin, M. (1997) Onset of speech after left hemispherectomy in a nine-year-old boy. *Brain* **120**, 159-182.

Learning Disability and Epilepsy: an Integrative Approach
Edited by Michael R. Trimble
© 2003 Clarius Press Ltd

6

Medial Temporal Lobe Structures in Epilepsy and Asperger Syndrome: Convergence of Evidence for Neural Circuitry Functions in Emotion

EKKEHART F. A. STAUFENBERG

Norwich Epilepsy Clinic, Department of Neurology
Norfolk & Norwich University Hospital NHS Trust
and School of Medicine, Health Policy and Practice
University of East Anglia, UK

INTRODUCTION

Asperger Syndrome (AS) forms part of the Pervasive Developmental Disorder category in international medical classificatory systems (see Box 1 and Box 2). Prompted by seminal work on the behavioural neurology of seizures of medial temporal lobe structures, studies of the neurodevelopmental biology and functional neurology of the syndrome have increasingly focussed on the roles of particular components of a neural network involved in emotion, namely the amygdala, its associated neural structures, and the hippocampus.

AS presents with a combination of symptoms and signs, which centre around pervasive, qualitative impairments in social relatedness and verbal and non-verbal communication, as well as interests, routines and repetitive behaviours. Three key hypotheses which seek to account for the syndrome's core deficit in social interactions include those of 'Theory of Mind'/ 'Social Intelligence', Executive Function, and the 'Central Coherence' Hypotheses. The former has been linked most explicitly to amygdala structures and neural circuitry based proposals, and encompass the capacity of an individual with AS to perceive and interpret other people's behaviour in terms of mental

BOX 1

Diagnostic Criteria for Asperger Syndrome / Asperger's Disorder according to International Classificatory and Research Manuals

ICD-10 (World Health Organisation, WHO, 1992)*

A   There is no clinically significant general delay in spoken or receptive language or cognitive development. Diagnosis requires that single words should have developed by 2 years of age or earlier, and that communicative phrases be used by 3 years of age or earlier. Self-help skills, adaptive behaviour, and curiosity about the environment during the first three years should be at a level consistent with normal intellectual development. However, motor milestones may be somewhat delayed and motor clumsiness is usual (although not a necessary diagnostic feature). Isolated special skills, often related to abnormal preoccupations, are common, but are not required for diagnosis.

B   There are qualitative abnormalities in reciprocal social interaction in at least two of the following areas (criteria as in autism):

(a) failure adequately to use eye-to-eye gaze, facial expression, body posture, and gesture to regulate social interaction

(b) failure to develop (in a manner appropriate to mental age, and despite ample opportunities) peer relationships that involve a mutual sharing of interest, activities and emotions

(c) lack of social-emotional reciprocity as shown by an impaired or deviant response to other people's emotions, or lack of modulation of behaviour according to social context; or a weak integration of social, emotional, and communicative behaviours

(d) lack of spontaneous seeking to share enjoyment, interests, or achievements with other people (e.g. a lack of showing, bringing, or pointing out to other people objects of interests to the individual)

C   The individual exhibits an unusually intense, circumscribed interest or restricted, repetitive, and stereotyped patterns of behaviour, interests, and activities in at least one of the following areas (criteria as for autism); however it would be less usual for these to include either motor mannerisms or preoccupations with part-objects or non-functional elements of play materials:

(a) an encompassing preoccupation with one or more stereotyped and restricted patterns of interest that are abnormal in their intensity and circumscribed nature though not in their content of focus

(b) apparently compulsive adherence to specific, non-functional routines or rituals

(c) stereotyped and repetitive motor mannerisms that involve either hand- or finger-flapping or –twisting, or complex whole-body movements

(d) preoccupations with part-objects or non-functional elements of play materials (such as their odour, the feel of their surface, or the noise or vibration that they generate)

D   The disorder is not attributable to the other varieties of pervasive developmental disorder: simple schizophrenia (F20.6); schizotypal disorder (F21); obsessive-compulsive disorder (F42); anankastic personality disorder (F60.5); reactive and disinhibited attachment disorders of childhood (F94.1 and F94.2, respectively).

* The criteria for Asperger Syndrome / Asperger's Disorder are currently being revised by Professor Fred Volkmar in cooperation with an international expert panel

---

BOX 2

Diagnostic Criteria for Asperger Syndrome / Asperger's Disorder according to International Classificatory and Research Manuals

DSM-IV Criteria (1994, American Psychiatric Association, APA)*

A Qualitative impairment in social interaction, as manifested by at least two of the following:

1   marked impairment in the use of multiple non-verbal behaviours such as eye-to-eye gaze, facial expression, body postures, and gesture to regulate social interaction

2   failure to develop peer relationships appropriate to developmental level

3   a lack of spontaneous seeking to share enjoyment, interests, or achievements with other people (e.g. by a lack of showing, bringing, or pointing out objects of interest to other people)

4   lack of social or emotional reciprocity

B Restricted repetitive and stereotyped patterns of behaviour, interests, and activities, as manifested by at least one of the following:

1   encompassing preoccupation with one or more stereotyped and restricted patterns of interest that is abnormal either in intensity or focus

2   apparently inflexible adherence to specific, non-functional routines or rituals

3   stereotyped and repetitive motor mannerisms (e.g. hand-or finger-flapping or –twisting, or complex whole-body movements)

4   persistent preoccupation with part of objects

C The disturbance causes clinically significant impairment in social, occupational, or other important areas of functioning.

D There is no clinically significant general delay in language (e.g. single words used by age 2 years, communicative phrases used by age 3 years).

E There is no clinically significant general delay in cognitive development or in the development of age-appropriate self-help skills, adaptive behaviour (other than in social interaction), and curiosity about the environment in childhood.

F Criteria are not met for another specific pervasive developmental disorder or schizophrenia.

* The criteria for Asperger Syndrome / Asperger's Disorder are currently being revised by Professor Fred Volkmar in cooperation with an international expert panel

---

states (emotions, beliefs, thoughts, intentions, desires), infer and / or predict their behaviours, and, as a result integrate within close social groups.

This chapter will introduce and review the current evidence that the amygdala, its extended neural substrates, and the hippocampus form part of a functionally continuous, neural network for the generation, mediation, and modulation of emotion. In its subsections, the chapter will summarise the studies of the structural, and functional neurobiological substrates informing the core deficits in AS (and autistic spectrum disorders), and finally conclude with a short review of theoretical and hypothetical neural circuitry models of autistic spectrum disorders and AS.

THE AMYGDALA AND ITS NEURAL CONNECTIONS

The amygdala is a key neuroanatomical substrate in the medial temporal lobe, involved both in the semiology of focal epilepsy syndromes, and proposed as the biological substrate for the autistic spectrum disorders' core qualitative impairments (Baron-Cohen *et al.*, 2000; Bechara, 2002).

Some 67 years after Broca's original description of the *'la grande lobe limbique'* (Broca, 1878), and 15 years after Papez' concept of a serially connected neural circuitry (hippocampal formation, mammillary body, [anterior] thalamic nuclei, the cortex of the gyrus cinguli, the hypothalamic

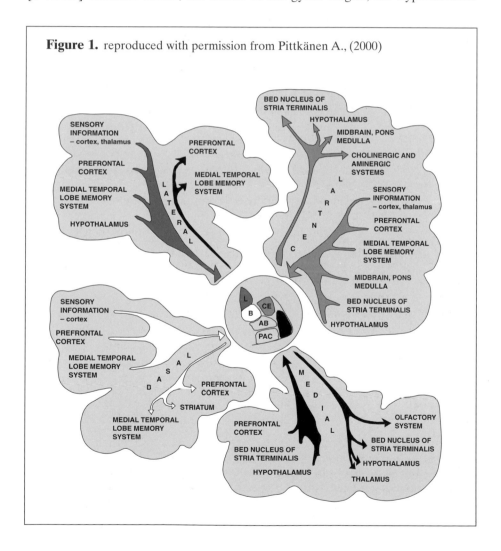

Figure 1. reproduced with permission from Pittkänen A., (2000)

region, and, for photic stimuli reception, the area striata) (Papez, 1937), Maclean (1952) first explicitly included the amygdala within the functional neuroanatomy of temporal lobe structures. Focal epilepsy seizure semiology has to date implicated the amygdala in primal functions such as aggression, anxiety, fear, appetitive and reproductive drives, somato-sensory perception (Eschle et al.,2002) and in simple partial seizures (SPS), with 'psychic auras' and auras of fear *(Commission on Classification and Terminology of the International League Against Epilepsy 1989)*.

The efferents and afferents of the amygdala are mostly reciprocal, direct or indirect neural connections with many brain structures including subcortical ones as part of the extended amygdala, and the prefrontal cortex (Heimer et al.,1997; Aggleton, 2000) (see Figure 1). The term 'extended amygdala' refers to the links between the amygdala (centro-medial nucleus) and subcortical structures such as the nucleus accumbens and the bed nucleus of the stria terminalis.

Histologically the amygdala is composed of subnuclei with distinct cytoarchitectural characteristics and neural connectivity. They can be subdivided into olfactory-, centromedial-, and basolateral neuronal groups (Gloor, 1997). The nuclei of the amygdala and 'extended amygdala' store, generate, mediate, and modulate a range of affective states, and contribute to their behavioural manifestations as part of direct and indirect, thalamic-prefrontal circuitries (Middleton, 2001).

Brown and Schäfer (Brown and Schäfer,1888), and particularly Klüver and Bucy (Klüver and Bucy, 1937) became alert to reproducible neurobehavioural changes after (bilateral) iatrogenic cat amygdala lesions which included loss of fear, changed species mating behaviour, and hyperphagia (including pica). They reported what they considered to be the key syndromal feature, namely the ablated cats' emotional indifference to sensory events, thus naming the syndrome 'psychic blindness'.

Further research confirmed the primate amygdala as the key neural substrate for the Klüver-Bucy Syndrome's core symptom of 'psychic blindness' (Pribram and Bagshaw,1953; Akert et al.,1961). This and other work (LeDoux, 1996; Rolls, 2000), outlined the presence of an extended neurofunctional integrity of amygdala circuitries (the extended amygdala) (Heimer et al., 1997), and led to the suggestion that 'psychic blindness' observed in the ablated cats was the neurobehavioural equivalent of human 'mind-blindness' (Baron-Cohen, 1995).

Bechara et al. (1995) reported that specific damage to the human amygdala produced an equivalent, qualitative and quantitative impairment of fear conditioning and emotional memory. Their data concurred with other findings of the amygdala's function in emotion memory (Buchel et al., 1998), which is maintained upon subliminal emotional conditioning stimuli (Morris et al., 1998), and remains unchanged irrespective of the presence of other stimuli designed to interfere with the direct right-sided thalamo-amygdala pathway involved in human emotional learning processes (Morris *et al.*, 1999).

Again, focal epilepsy research paradigms inform much of the current understanding on the amygdala's neuroplasticity, and are now being applied to pervasive neurodevelopmental disorders including AS (Baron-Cohen *et al.*, 2000). Amygdala neuroplasticity manifests in both neural cytoarchitecture and synaptic restructuring, leading to short-term and long-term electrochemical potentiation (Gloor, 1997), and may be studied in the experimental model of kindling (Goddard *et al.*, 1969).

Hippocampal and Amygdala
– functional connectivity with other brain regions –

Comparative neuroanatomy confirms that the brain's developmental evolution across species leads to individual brain regions acquiring and integrating increasingly complex functions (Damasio, 1995). Whilst some key neurobehavioural functions are preferentially lateralised to one or the other cerebral hemisphere, three phylogenetically distinct interhemispheric connections ensure transfer of certain information, namely the corpus callosum, the anterior commissures, and the hippocampal commissures (Demeter *et al.*, 1990).

The corpus callosum incorporates, amongst others, diverse limbic system axons, and includes the amygdala's major projections to the orbital frontal cortex (OFC; Amaral *et al.*, 1984). The anterior commissure ensures transhemispheric communication for the key structures of the limbic system. In primates, the hippocampal commissure carries interhemispheric connections via a dorsal pathway to the opposite hippocampus (Demeter *et al.*, 1990), and is the neural substrate for the development from (unilateral) simple partial to (bilateral) complex partial seizures in focal (localisation-related) epilepsy syndromes (Wilson *et al.*, 1990).

The amygdala's cortico-subcortical projections, however, largely terminate ipsilaterally, and only a small proportion reach the contralateral medial temporal lobe and they do not connect with the contralateral amygdala at all (Demeter *et al.*, 1990). Their diversification goes parallel to the increased diversification in social cognition and behaviours associated with the evolutionary development of species, with relatively limited neural afferents (and efferents) in the cat , compared with those in macaque amygdala, and humans (Shammah-Lagnado *et al.*, 2001; Heimer *et al.*, 1997).

This lack of significant interhemispheric connectivity for both the hippocampus or amygdala (Engel and Shewmon, 1991) is pertinent to the current hypothesis that both emotional tone and affect are lateralised to the right hemisphere and may relate largely to ipsihemispheric specialised neural structures, comparable to the lateralisation of verbal and spatial memory (Amaral *et al.*, 1984; Demeter *et al.*, 1990).

Predominant right ipsilateral amygdala connectivity has been considered important for autistic spectrum disorders in terms of dysfunctional inter-hemispheric information transfer between the medial temporal lobes (Dawson *et al.*, 1998). This includes the possibility of altered interhemispheric lateralisation, a putative transfer dysfunction accounting for the increased prevalence of 'non-right handedness' in autistic spectrum disorders (Gillberg, 1983), and lower left hemispheric regional cerebral blood flow overall in relation to sensorimotor and language functions in autism (Chiron *et al.*, 1995), as well as right hemisphere mediated prosodic abnormalities.

The Amygdala and neural mechanism of emotion
– current perspectives –

The early neuroanatomical studies on amygdala function led to several research directions, including electrostimulation, neurotransmitter, and neuroradiological ones. The low threshold susceptibility to electric stimulation of the hippocampus CA1 region, and the central nucleus of the amygdala (Schwartzkroin and McIntyre, 1997), allowed specific electrostimulation studies of their acute and chronic neurophysiological changes to be undertaken (Engel and Shewmon, 1991; McNamara *et al.*, 1997).

Penfield and colleagues used amygdala electrostimulation, and helped dispel the view, held up to that time, of the hypothalamus as 'the centre of the brain's emotional system' (LeDoux, 2000). The work delineated specific seizure semiologies elicited in humans under local anaesthetic, and still forms the basis for current seizure classifications. They described 'experiential mental phenomena' such as auditory, visual, combined visual and auditory, and unclassified experiences such as dreams, flashbacks, déjà vu and déjà entendu (Penfield and Rasmussen, 1957).

Their seminal research anticipated convergent evidence for the amygdala as the core neural substrate in the homeostasis of emotional tone, and affective changes (Halgren, *et al.*, 1978; Schwartzkroin and McIntyre, 1997), which in turn informed research of the functions of other brain circuits in emotion based behaviours which are not considered here any further (but see Fuster, 1997; Lichter and Cummings, 2001).

Neurotransmitter based research of the role of the amygdala in emotion focused largely on the $GABA_A$/benzodiazepine (BZPs) receptor complex, notwithstanding other areas in the brain in which benzodiazepines may exert their anxiolytic effects such as the dorsal hippocampus, dorsal and median raphe nuclei and the dorsal periaqueductal grey (Fine, 2000). The amygdala has the highest density for BZP binding sites in the brain (Niehoff and Kuhar, 1983) and specifically in the limbic system (Onoe *et al.*,1996).

In the amygdala, abolition of fear responses takes place when the structure is lesioned (File *et al.*, 1998). Fear and anxiety can be induced by electrical stimulation (Feindel and Penfield,1954), which are accompanied by regional blood flow changes (Zald and Pardo,1997). Further, the amygdala can modify hippocampal long-term memory storage via arousal-state-dependent amygdala functioning (Cahil, 2000). A reduction of the firing rate of amygdaloid neurons, with associated anxiolytic effects when benzodiazepines are injected directly into rat amygdala is particularly prominent if targeting the basolateral nuclear complex (Gonzalez *et al.*, 1996).

Hence the key modulatory role of the amygdala in emotion works at least in part via a 'central fear system involved in both the expression and acquisition of conditioned and unconditioned fear' and associated neurobehavioural changes, particularly in the case of 'conditioned aversive memory involving fear and anxiety' (Davis *et al.*, 1994).

This learning process is prevented by amygdala inactivation (Muller *et al.*, 1997), if the inactivation takes place prior to, but *not after* the learning event (Wilensky *et al.*, 2000), thereby suggesting that the amygdala is essential for adaptive fear learning, and does not modulate its own learning after the event. Whether these observations are relevant to the high harm avoidance anxiety traits recorded in AS (Soderstrom *et al.*, 2002) remains to be explored, bearing in mind the evidence that neural transmission of emotion preferentially involves thalamo-amygdala connections with slower conditioning of the cortical pathway (Quirk *et al.*,1997), possible preferential use of a designated right amygdala–specific projection pathway (Morris *et al.*, 1999), and amygdala neuroplasticity initially affecting the subcortical rather than the thalamic pathways (LeDoux ,1996).

In summary, the study of the amygdala's specific role in the development of emotion, the maintenance of emotional traits and affective states, and its contributions in their generation, mediation and modulation are only beginning to emerge. The (extended) amygdala's place in emotional control involves specific nuclear groups which work as a functionally unitary circuitry with extensive excitatory efferent and reciprocal afferent connections essential to acquisition and expression of emotion as found in anxiety and fear paradigms.

These functions may be contingently responsive to specific social stimuli, including sociovisual ones (Thomas *et al.*, 2001), and mediate and modulate voluntary, goal-directed associative behaviours whose absence has been shown to be incompatible with an organism's survival (Kling and Brothers, 1992; Gallagher, 2000), or maintenance of social status within a social group (Barton and Dunbar, 1997).

Asperger Syndrome, Theory of Mind /'Social Intelligence', Central Coherence, and Executive Function

Perhaps prompted by Kanner's original concept that children with autism have 'inborn disturbances of affective contact' (Kanner, 1943), Hans Asperger's seminal work (Asperger, 1943) and a hypothesis that 'psychic blindness' in cats may be equivalent to 'mindblindness' in humans, research into the neurobiological basis of autistic syndromes and AS has evolved (Gillberg, 2000a,b). This includes the search for greater clarification, via genetic modelling (Rutter et al., 1993), of existing genetic predisposing factors (Volkmar et al., 1993b).

A 'multiple primary deficit model' of autism (Minshew et al., 1997), compatible with a neural network hypothesis with regards to subcortical and cortical connectivities, inherent in the amygdadalo-hippocampal-thalamo-prefrontal cortical circuitries, has also been postulated (Gustafsson, 1997).

With regard to the qualitative impairments in AS (see Box 1), there are currently three, potentially complementary hypotheses:

(a) the 'Meta-Representational theory', which is now commonly being referred to by a term originating from primate research, namely the 'Theory of Mind' (ToM),

(b) the 'Central Coherence Theory', and

(c) the 'Executive Function Theory'.

Meta-Representational Theory

The central tenet of the 'Meta-representational Theory' or 'Theory of Mind'(ToM), originally revolved around the concept of a neurobiological disorder of empathy. Others developed the concept of qualitative (and quantitative) impairments (Wing and Gould, 1979), and a deficit in the capacity to conceive of other people's mental states (Frith, 1989; Baron-Cohen, 1990), with some variations dependent on the severity of co-existing cognitive impairment (Baron-Cohen, 1995).

The ToM has been particularly considered in relation to pervasive socialisation, and communication difficulties, manifesting at earlier developmental milestones via abnormalities in protoimperative and protodeclarative pointing, showing of objects, and eye-gaze to regulate contact (Stone et al., 1997).

The neural basis of the ToM and 'Social Intelligence' (Baron-Cohen et al., 2000) has been linked to the amygdala, the orbito-frontal cortex, and the superior temporal gyrus, all of which have been linked to the core deficits in autism (Kling and Brothers, 1992; Stuss et al., 2002).

Central Coherence Theory

The term 'Central Coherence' denotes a person's cognitive style on a hypothesised spectrum ranging from 'weak' to 'strong'. A person with 'weak' Central Coherence is said to have a cognitive style characterised by fragmentation of information into its constitutent parts, and difficulties in switching from detail to conceptualised inferential thinking patterns. Those said to demonstrate 'strong' Central Coherence show superior associative, 'gist' cognitive styles.

AS and high functioning autistic individuals perform at the 'weak' Central Coherence spectrum of the continuum, as shown by superior skills in the 'Embedded Figures Test' (Jolliffe and Baron-Cohen, 1997), counting abilities (Jarrold and Russell, 1997), bloc design subtests (Frith, 1989), and relatively lower scores on the object assembly subtest (Ehlers *et al.*, 1997).

Executive Function Theory

The Executive Function Theory proposes that the syndromes' qualitative impairments relate to deficits in a capacity to perform tasks such as initiation of action, planning, execution of purposive, sequential actions, self-regulation and reflection, and volition (Lezak, 1995). The prefrontal cortex, and its orbital-frontal area, which is linked particulary to the amygdala (LeDoux, 1996), is proposed as the neural substrate for these executive functions (Lichter and Cummings, 2001).

Executive functions have been shown to be impaired in autistic spectrum disorders (Courchesne *et al.*, 1994), especially in AS (Ozonoff and Miller, 1996), and high functioning autism (Nydén *et al.*, 1999). ADHD, and dyslexia differ from normal controls in their executive function profile, but not between each other (Nydén *et al.*, 1999), leaving the question of the presence or not of specific executive dysfunction in Asperger's Syndrome open to further enquiry.

Amygdala structures in Asperger Syndrome
– neurofunctional substrates of social impairments –

The previous sections of this chapter have summarised an array of complex neurobehavioural functions involving the amygdala as the centre of a cortico-subcortical neural circuitry which generates, mediates and modulates emotion and aspects of social behaviours, such as 'making sense of verbal and non-verbal dimensions, decoding and the integration of perceptual features from other individuals, and the modulation and generation of the social context's appropriate emotional tone, affective state, cognitive - , motor - , autonomic - , and other behavioural responses' (Aggleton, 1993).

Comparative evolutionary research (Price *et al.*, 1987) has shown, for higher primates, increasing amygdala efferent and afferent ramifications as cortical brain regions enlarge with complex social interactions (Young *et al.*, 1994). The data show a parallel evolution of amygdala-based neurons responsive to faces in very young macaques and humans, absent or less developed in other primates (Dolan, 2000).

In humans, the first study to examine developmental differences in amygdala responses to facial fear expressions using a controlled fMRI study design (Thomas *et al.*, 2001) found the left amygdala of adults to respond more to fear than neutral facial emotion, that the amygdala of children showed more signal attenuation for neutral but not fear expressions, with no lateral differentiation, and reported a gender-specific interaction. The amygdala function of boys but not girls habituated substantially more to facial fear expressions. The authors did not comment specifically on the presence or otherwise of lateralised differences, or on the intellectual ability levels of their subjects. However, their findings are compatible with similar gender effects reported in normal children and young people (Gidd *et al.*, 1996). They are also in keeping with neurostructural studies in high functioning autistic study populations (Aylward *et al.*, 1999) and metabolite studies using 1-H Spectroscopy, which have revealed significantly reduced concentrations of N-acetyl-aspartate [NAA], a marker of neuronal integrity, in right versus left amygdala-hippocampal structures in autistic but not normal children (Otsuka *et al.*, 1999). Whether these results reflect neuronal dysfunction and or immaturity or are secondary to dysfunction of neuronal circuitries or functional networks remains uncertain. The significance of these data, however, require further, larger scale and comprehensive study designs to better control for contributory variables which could lead to hitherto unrecognised interactions.

With regard to the ToM, or 'social intelligence', Kling (Kling *et al.*, 1972; Kling and Brothers, 1992) comprehensively reviewed the evidence for and against the neurofunctional involvement of the amygdala. Their amygdala lesioned vervets and rhesus monkeys were unable to survive when returned to their group because they failed to interact socially (no affiliation, eg grooming, or aggression), preferred social withdrawal, and often succumbed to their peers' attacks. The acquired deficit in social reciprocity remained chronic in studies where lesions were more circumscribed (Bachevalier, 1991), or if the lesion included the amygdala, hippocampus, entorhinal and perirhinal cortices (Bachevalier, 1994) whilst amygdala–(or hippocampus–) *only* lesions showed weaker phenotypic deficits over time

Their study design, however, did not permit the examination of amygdala neuroplasticity to possibly account for the progressive weakening of the social behaviour deficits in amygdala–only lesions. Yet results are consistent with the loss of social status reported for amygdalectomised 'head' monkeys (Adolphs and Tranel, 2000), and the resulting disruption of the entire group's social structure (Rosvold *et al.*, 1954).

Human functional neuroradiological data, however, do not converge similarly. The single study, which detected amygdala activation, used an *eye-gaze* only test image paradigm (e.g. not whole face expression) to assess 'social intelligence'(Baron-Cohen *et al.*, 1999), a finding which converges with the amygdala's previously confirmed specific neural responsiveness to emotional information conveyed by eye gaze (Kawashima *et al.*, 1999). Most other studies have used whole face emotional expression test image paradigms, and report a lack of amygdala activation in serial fMRIs (Fletcher *et al.*, 1995; Brunet *et al.*, 2000; Gallagher *et al.*, 2000; Vogeley *et al.*, 2001).

Other data show a significant role of the amygdala in aversive conditioning in both rodents, monkeys and healthy human volunteers (Lamprecht and Dudai, 2000). The models include Hare-Psychopathy (Hare and Quinn, 1971), augmentation of the startle reflex (Levenston *et al.*, 2000), recognition of fearful expressions in defensive – but not offensive - aggression in 'in vivo' focal epilepsy syndromes (Kalynchuk *et al.*, 1999), and in aggression found in that small proportion of medial temporal lobe epilepsy patients which are associated with more widespread dual brain pathology of left hemispheric encephalitic origin (van Elst, 2002). All these studies implicitly or explicitly acknowledge the important role of other brain regions in addition to the amygdala, such as the hippocampus (Stuss *et al.*, 2002), and the projections with the prefrontal cortex (Lichter and Cummings, 2001) in these behaviours.

At a cytoarchitectural level, the neural substrates for facial emotional expressivity have been mapped to designated amygdala 'face neurons' with afferent connections from other 'face cells' in the inferior temporal cortex and superior temporal sulcus (Brothers *et al.*, 1990). The firing rate of these neurones changes only as emotional facial expressivity changes, but not during pure (static) face recognition tasks (Adolphs and Tranel, 2000; Dolan, 2000; Rolls, 2000).

In summary the amygdala's specific role within the neural circuitry involved with social functioning, emotion, and memory appears – on current evidence – to lie with the perception of emotional and affective changes both within the individual, and within the environment.

Neurophysiological and focal epilepsy syndrome research, comparative neuroanatomical, neurodevelopmental, neuropsychological, and forensic neuropsychiatric evidence support this specific mediating, and modulating amygdala role, using both emotional facial expressivity (but not still photographs to measure pure facial recognition), and classical and operant fear conditioning contingency study designs. Dysfunction of these neural circuitries, both neurodevelopmental (Rolls, 2000; Blair *et al.*, 2001), or acquired (Blair and Cipolotti, 2000), will disadvantage the individual organism thus affected by way of acquired social difficulties and /or violations of social norms (Berthoz *et al.*, 2002). Explanatory hypotheses of dysfunctions of neural circuitries in autistic spectrum disorders have been proposed using parallel network simulation in mathematical models, and cortical mapping paradigms (Gustafsson, 1997; Minshew *et al.*, 1997), but require further examination.

Clinical Case

The complex neurofunctional circuitry involved in Asperger Syndrome has recently been discussed in a pre- versus post right amygdalo-hippocampectomy case for mesial temporal sclerosis and AS (Staufenberg, for publication), which lead the authors to hypothesis an 'Amygdala-mediated Neuroinhibition Effect' (ANE).

Case History

A man of average IQ, with right Mesial Temporal Sclerosis (MTS), a focal (local-isation-related) epilepsy syndrome with simple and complex partial seizures, at times with secondary generalisation, and AS underwent complete right-sided amygdalo-hippocampectomy, and anterior temporal lobectomy.

The life-long clinical seizures stopped despite ongoing pathological EEG with spikes and spike/wave dysrrhythmias. Over the 36 months, since the epilepsy surgery, the man's qualitative impairments especially in the domains of social reciprocity, communication (verbal and non-verbal) including prosody, and repetitive repertoire have undergone significant improvements as measured by pre - versus post-neurosurgery scores on the Autism Diagnostic Interview – revised (ADI-R, 3rd edition; Lord *et al.*, 1994), the ASDI (Gillberg *et al.*, 2001), clinical criteria (Box 3; Gillberg and Ehlers, 1998), and international classifica-tory systems (Leekam *et al.*, 2000), in the absence of significant alteration of verbal or non-verbal memory process on psychometry (Dupont *et al.*, 2002).

The authors propose an 'Amygdala-mediated Emotion Gate' (AEG), which manifests post-amygdalo-hippocampectomy as a 'Neurobehavioural Release Effect' (NRE). This is a disinhibitory neural function, possibly acting via the right amygdala's specific neural pathways which mediates unconscious and conscious emotional learning (Morris *et al.*, 1998), and subliminal fear signals (Morris *et al.*, 1999). The 'NRE' would be compatible with a postulated increase in the threshold of a sensory signal necessary to trigger emotional responses in autistic disorders (Aggleton, 1992), and the reported postencephalopathic resolution of autistic symtomatologies in children (DeLong *et al.*, 1981). The authors considered the adaptive changes post-neurosurgically in the context of a defective sensorimotor gating mechanism, postulated for the fronto-striatal pathways, in AS (McAlonan *et al.*, 2002) which form part of a wider neural network involved in autistic spectrum disorder core deficits.

BOX 3

Diagnostic Criteria for Asperger Syndrome / Asperger's Disorder according to International Classificatory and Research Manuals

Gillberg & Gillberg's (1989) diagnostic criteria, revised (Gillberg, 1991)

1   Social Impairment (extreme egocentricity)

(at least two of the following):

(a) Inability to interact with peers

(b) Lack of desire to interact with peers

(c) Lack of appreciation of social cues

(d) Socially and emotionally inappropriate behaviour

2   Narrow interest

(at least one of the following):

(a) Exclusion of other activities

(b) Repetitive adherence

(c) More rote than meaning

3   Repetitive routines

(at least one of the following):

(a) on self, in aspects of life

(b) on others

4   Speech and language peculiarities

(at least three of the following):

(a) Delayed development

(b) Superficially perfect expressive language

(c) Formal pedantic language

(d) Odd prosody, peculiar voice characteristics

(e) Impairment of comprehension including misinterpretations of literal/implied meanings

5   Non-verbal communication problems

(a) Limited use of gestures

(b) Clumsy/gauche body language

(c) Limited facial expression

(d) Inappropriate expression

(e) Peculiar, stiff gaze

6   Motor clumsiness

(a) Poor performance on neuro-developmental examination

ASPERGER'S SYNDROME, NEURAL AND BEHAVIOURAL PLASTICITY
- SUMMARY AND CONCLUSION -

The complex nature of the behavioural phenotypes associated with autistic spectrum disorders is undisputed (Gillberg., 2000b). They include the greater prevalence of males in autistic populations, particularly amongst those with higher IQ levels (Volkmar *et al.*, 1993a), higher autism scores on early social developmental ratings (McLennan *et al.*, 1993), very high risk for (often focal, localisation-related) cryptogenic epilepsy syndromes (Gillberg and Coleman, 2000) with their own neuropsychiatric complications (Trimble and Schmitz, 2002), and the measurable presence in AS of discrete personality trait ratings. These are especially high for 'harm avoidance', and '(social) anxiety traits', and low for 'self-directedness' and 'cooperativeness' scores (Soderstrom *et al.*, 2002).

Current models of the behavioural neurology of the autistic spectrum and AS provide support for a central deficit in higher-order cognitive functions localized at multiple levels within a parallel processing based cortico-subcortical neural axis (Alexander *et al.* 1990; Lichter and Cummings 2001). Postulated 'multiple primary deficits' in these neural networks are currently being explored with regard to the neurobiology of autistic disorders and AS.

Prompted by focal (localisation-related) epilepsy syndrome based research, the amygdala and its affiliate structures are now known to represent a key nodal circuitry which manages the generation, mediation and modulation of emotion and emotional learning, and the integration of sensory with neurocognitive -, motor -, somatosensory, and autonomic behaviours, often via subliminal learning processes (Morris *et al.*, 1998). The (extended) amygdala's extensive, reciprocal or unidirectional neural connectivity with so many brain regions reflect its pivotal functions (Pitkänen, 2000).

These interactive, dynamic neuroregulatory amydala functions subserve 'the regulation of behaviours via knowledge of the emotional responses and intentions ('Theory of Mind / Social intelligence') of others' (Brothers, 1995), and are selectively affected by amygdala damage when cognitive (thinking) skills remain intact (Barton and Aggleton, 2000). The incapacity, clinically, of AS probands to relay emotional experiences, rather than reflecting rote memory-based descriptions of emotions, seems an apposite observation in this context.

Rare cases of acquired or congenital amygdala lesions have provided some further insight into current hypotheses in autistic spectrum disorders (Adolphs *et al.*,1998). Bilateral stereotactic amygdala damage (Scott *et al.*, 1997), congenital bilateral calcification of the amygdala (Adolphs *et al.*, 1995), and post-encephalitic amygdala damage (Broks *et al.*, 1998) all adversely affect social affiliation, social learning, social interpersonal boundaries, or produce deficits in 'social judgement of approachability and trustworthiness from faces of unfamiliar people' (Adolphs *et al.*, 1998). Similarly mesial temporal lobe sclerosis (MTS) of the right amygdalo-hippocampal structures adversely affects prosodic function of language relating to right hemisphere lateralised intonation, stress, rhythm, and tempo in both children (Bell *et al.*, 1990), and adults (Ross, 1993).

Damasio (Damasio and Maurer, 1978) proposed a bilateral cerebral neural network that could account for the symptoms and signs of autistic disorders, and ongoing research continues to enhance the evidence for a network supporting current neurocognitive hypotheses for the core impairments in autistic disorders including AS (Brothers, 1995; Baron-Cohen *et al.*, 1999).

Bilateral damage, specifically to the amygdala (Bauman and Kemper, 1993), and unilateral neuropatholgogy have been implicated in social and communication deficits (Fein *et al.*, 1987), empathy (Brothers, 1989), in the difficulties to appropriately decode the emotional significance of incoming stimuli and assigning them appropriate motivational importance (Fotheringham, 1991). Theories also consider the nature of the neurofunctional connectivity of the amygdala with the prefrontal cortex (Baron-Cohen *et al.*, 1999).

The central role of the amygdala has recently been further highlighted by targeted functional imaging studies in autistic populations by Piven *et al.*, (1998), which revoked the same group's earlier findings (Piven *et al.*, 1997) of predominantly hippocampal abnormalities.

The evidence for lateralisation of neurofunction in autistic disorders requires further specific study designs in autistic spectrum disorders and Asperger Syndrome. However, findings of right hemisphere lateralisation of neurodysfunction and a generalised decrease in perfusion (George *et al.*,1992), is possibly related to neuromaturational processes in the prefrontal cortical regions of autistic children (Zilbovicius *et al.*, 1995). The exploration of such networks may lead, also, to greater clarity about the well established link of autistic disorders and AS with the neurobiology of affective and other neuropsychiatric disorders (Staufenberg, 1994).

Taking all of above information and hypotheses together, the amygdala nuclei seem to encompass critical neuromodulatory functions for the retrieval of socially relevant knowledge on the basis of facial and other sensory information, including, in some children with AS, enhancement of processing skills of the affective components of specific musical skills (Heaton *et al.*, 1999).

The focal (localisation-related) epilepsy models of medial temporal lobe structures confirm a cytoarchitecture and projection pathway-based maturational and developmental neuroplasticity (Stefan, 1999), which has a capacity to undergo neuromaturational processes in response to acute or chronic neuropathological stimuli including those implicated in the aetiopathogenesis of autistic spectrum disorders and AS. These factors include intrauterine, in particular second trimester pathology (Coleman, 1994; Torrey *et al.*, 1975), perinatal (rare), and post-natal (Kemper and Bauman, 1998) acquired, or developmental neuropathology (Webster *et al.*, 1991).

With regard to the dynamic interaction of the amygdala with other brain regions, Aggleton recognised that the emotional changes following bilateral amygdala lesions do not necessarily determine a complete lack of emotional responsivity. They may rather relate to an increase in the threshold of a sensory signal necessary to trigger the emotional responses (Aggleton, 1992).

The recent renaissance of a focal (localisation-related) epilepsy syndrome-based iatrogenic lesion approach to elicit neural circuitry-based functions in emotion (Pitkänen *et al.*, 1998) may amplify theoretical mathematical models of parallel processes, which suggest *'a multiple primary deficit model [of high functioning autism]... in which the deficit pattern within and across domains is reflective of the complexity of the information processing demands, ...'* (Cohen, 1994). Amongst others, careful circumscribed iatrogenic or anecdotal lesion-based data may examine an earlier neurophysiological characterisation of autism as *'a late information processing disorder which spares early information processing'* (Gillberg *et al.*, 2001) in the context of modern neurofunctional hypotheses generated by ongoing research in epilepsy syndromes.

REFERENCES

Adolphs, R. and Tranel, D. (2000). Emotion, recognition, and the human amygdala. In: J.P. Aggleton (Ed.), *The Amygdala – A Functional Analysis*. Oxford University Press. Oxford, pp 587-630.

Adolphs, R., Tranel, D. and Damasio, A.R. (1998). The human amygdala in social judgement. *Nature* **393**, 470-474.

Adolphs, R., Tranel, D., Damasio, H. and Damasio, H.R. (1995). Fear and the human amygdala. *J Neurosci* **15**, 5879-5891.

Aggleton, J.P. (1992). The functional effects of amygdala lesions in humans: a comparison with findings from monkeys. In: Aggleton, J.P. (Ed), *The Amygdala: Neurobiological Aspects of Emotion, Memory, and Dysfunction*. Wiley-Liss, New York, pp. 485-503.

Aggleton, J.P. (1993). The contribution of the amygdala to normal and abnormal emotional states. *Trends Neurosci* **16**, 328-333.

Aggleton , J.P. (2000). The amygdala – what's happened in the last decade? In: Aggleton, J.P. (Ed). The Amygdala – A Functional Analysis. Oxford University Press, Oxford, pp. 1-30.

Akert, K., Gruesen, R.A., Woolsey, C.N. and Meyer, D.R. (1961). Klüver-Bucy Syndrome in monkeys with neocortical ablations of temporal lobe. *Brain* **84**, 480-497.

Alexander G.E., Crutcher, M.D. and DeLong, M.R. (1990). Basal ganglia-thalamo-cortical circuits: parallel substrates for motor, oculomotor, 'prefrontal', and 'limbic' functions. *Prog Brain Res* **85**, 119-146.

Amaral, D.G., Insausti, R. and Cowan, W.M. (1984). The commissural connections of the monkey hippocampal formation. *J Comp Neurol* **224**, 307-336.

Asperger, H. (1943). *Die autistischen Psychopathen im Kindesalter.* PhD Thesis, University Medical School, Vienna.

Aylward, E.H., Minshaw, N.J., Goldstein, G., Honeycutt, N.A., Augustine, M., Yates, K.O., Barta, P.-E., Parkson, G..D. *et al.* (1999). MRI volumes of amygdala and hippocampus in non-mentally retarded autistic adolescents and adults. *Neurology* **53**, 2145-2150.

Bachevalier, J. (1991). An animal model for childhood autism: memory loss and socioemotional disturbances following neonatal damage to the limbic system in monkeys. In: Tamminga. C., Schulz, S. (Eds), *Advances in Neuropsychiatric Psychopharmacology.* Raven Press, New York, pp. 129-140.

Bachevalier, J. (1994). Medial temporal lobe structures and autism: a review of clinical and experimental findings. *Neuropsychologia* **32**, 627-648.

Bachevalier J. (2000). The amygdala, social behaviour, and autism. In Aggleton J.P. (Ed.). *The Amygdala – A Functional Analysis.* Oxford University Press, Oxford, pp 509-544.

Baron-Cohen, S. (1990). Autism: a specific cognitive disorder of 'mind-blindness". *Intern Rev Psychiatry* **2**, 81-90.

Baron-Cohen, S. (1995). *Mind Blindness. An Essay on Autism and Theory of mind.* MIT Press, Cambridge, Mass, USA.

Baron-Cohen, S., Ring, H.A., Bullmore, E.T., Wheelwright, S., Ashwin, C. and Williams, S.C.R. (2000). The amygdala theory of autism. *Neurosci Biobehav Rev*, **24**, 355-364.

Baron-Cohen, S., Ring, H.A., Wheelwright, S., Bullmore, E.T., Brammer, M.J., Simmons, A. and Williams, S.C.R. (1999). Social intelligence in the normal and autistic brain: an fMRI study. *Eur J Neurosci* **11**, 1891-1898.

Barton, R.A. and Aggleton, J.P. (2000). Primate evolution and the amygdala. In: Aggleton, J.P. (Ed), *The Amgydala – A Functional Analysis.* Oxford University Press, Oxford, pp. 479-508.

Barton, R.A. and Dunbar, R.I.M. (1997). Evolution of the social brain. In: Whiten, A. and Byrne, R.W. (Eds), *Machiavellian Intelligence II.* Cambridge University Press, Cambridge, pp. 240-263.

Bauman,A.L. and Kemper, T.L. (1993). Cytoarchitectonic changes in the brain of people with autism. In: Bauman, A.L. and Kemper, T.L. (Eds), *The Neurobiology of Autism.* John Hopkins Press, Baltimore, pp. 119-145.

Bechara, A. (2002). The neurology of social cognition. Editorial. *Brain* **125**, 1673-1675.

Bechara, A., Tranel, D., Damasio, H., Adolphs, R., Rockland, C. and Damasio, A.R. (1995). Double dissociation of conditioning and declarative knowledge relative to the amygdala and hippocampus in humans. *Science* **269**, 1115-1118.

Bell, W.L., Davis, D.L., Morgan-Fisher, A. and Ross, E.D. (1990). Acquired aprosodia in children. *J Child Neurol* **5**, 19-26.

Berthoz, S., Armony, J.L., Blair, R.J.R. and Dolan, R.J. (2002). An fMRI study of intentional and unintentional (embarrassing) violations of social norms. *Brain* **125**, 1696-1708.

Blair, R.J. and Cipolotti, L. (2000). Impaired social response reversal: a case of 'acquired sociopathy'. *Brain* **123**, 1122-1141.

Blair, R.J., Colledge, E., Murray, L. and Mitchell, D.G. (2001). A selective impairment in the processing of sad and fearful expressions in children with psychopathic tendencies. *J Abnorm Child Psychol* **29**, 491-498.

Broca, P. (1878). Anatomie comparée des circonvolutions cérébrales. La grande lobe limbique et la scisssure limbique dans le série des mammifères. *Rev Anthropol*, **21**, 385-498.

Broks, P., Young, A.W., Maratos, E.J., Coffey, P.J., Calder, A.J., Isaac, C.L., Mayes, A.R., Hodges, J.R., Montaldi, D., Cezayirli, E., Roberts, N. and Hadley, D. (1998). Face processing impairments after encephalitis: amygdala damage and recognition of fear. *Neuropsychologia* **36**, 59-70.

Brothers, L. (1989). A biological perspective on empathy. *Am J Psychiatry* **146**, 10-19.

Brothers, L. (1995). Neurophysiology of the perception of intention by primates. In: Gazzaniga, M.S. (Ed), *The Cognitive Neurosciences*. MIT Press, Cambridge, Mass, pp. 1107-1117.

Brothers, L., Ring, B. and Kling, A. (1990). Response of neurons in the macaque amygdala to complex social stimuli. *Behav Brain Res* **41**, 199-213.

Brown, S. and Schäfer, A. (1888). An investigation in the functions of the occipital and temporal lobes of the monkey's brain. *Philosophical Transactions of the Royal Society of London*, Series B, **179**, 303-327.

Brunet, E., Sarfati, Y., Hardy-Bayle, M.C. and Decety J. (2000). A PET investigation of the attribution of intentions with a nonverbal task. *Neuroimage* **11**, 157-166.

Buchel, C., Morris, J., Dolan, R.J. and Friston, K.J. (1998). Brain systems mediating aversive conditioning: an event-related fMRI study. *Neuron* **20**, 947-957.

Cahill, L. (2000) Modulation of long term memory storage in humans by emotional arousal: adrenergic activation and the amygdala. In: Aggleton, J.P. (Ed), *The Amygdala – A Functional Analysis*. Oxford University Press, Oxford, pp. 426-445.

Chiron, C., Leboyer, M., Leon, F., Jambaque, I., Nuttin, C. and Syrot, A. (1995). SPECT of the brain in childhood autism: evidence for a lack of normal hemispheric asymmetry. *Dev Med Child Neurol* **37**, 849-860.

Cohen, I.L. (1994). An artificial neural analogue of learning in autism. *Biol Psychiatry* **36**, 5-20.

Coleman, M. (1994). Second trimester of gestation: a time of risk for classical autism? *Dev Brain Dysfunction* **7**, 104-109.

Commission on Classification and Terminology of the International League Against Epilepsy (1989). A revised proposal for the classification of epilepsy and epileptic syndromes. *Epilepsia* **30**, 268-278.

Courchesne, E., Townsend, J.P., Akshoomoff, N..A., Yeung-Courchesne, R., Press, G.A., Murakami, J.W., Lincoln, A.J., James, H.E. and Saitoh, O. (1994). A new finding: Impairment in shifting attention in autistic and cerebellar patients. In: Broman, S.H. and Grafman, J. (Eds), *Atypical Cognitive Deficits in Developmental Disorders: Implications for Brain Function*. Erlbaum, Hillsdale, N.J. pp. 101-137.

Damasio, A.R. (1995). *Descartes' Error: Emotion, Reason and the Human Brain*. Picador, London.

Damasio, A.R. and Maurer, R.G. (1978). A neurological model for childhood autism. *Arch Neurol* **35**, 777-786.

Davis, M., Hitchcock, J.M., Bowers, M.B. Berridge, C.W., Melia, K.R. and Roth R.H. (1994). Stress-induced activation of prefrontal cortex dopamine turnover: blockade by lesions of the amygdala. *Brain Res* **664**, 207-210.

Dawson, G., Meltzoff, A.N., Osterling, J. and Rinaldi, J. (1998). Neuropsychological correlates of early symptoms of autism. *Child Dev* **69**, 1276-1285.

DeLong, G.R. Bean, S.C. and Brown, F.R. (1981). Acquired reversible autistic syndrome in acute encephalopathic illness children. *Arch Neurol* **38**, 191-194.

Demeter, D., Rosene, D.L. and Van Hoesen, G.W. (1990). Fields of origins and pathways of the interhemispheric commisures in the temporal lobe of macaques. *J Comp Neurol* **302**, 29f.

Dolan, R.J. (2000). Functional neuroimaging of the amygdala during emotional processing and learning. In: Aggleton, J.P. (Ed), *The Amygdala – A Functional Analysis.* Oxford University Press, Oxford, pp. 631-654.

Dupont, S., Samson, Y., Van de Moortele, P.-F., Poline, J.B., Hasboun, D., Le Bihan, D. and Baulac, M. (2002). Bilateral hemispheric alteration of memory processes in right medial temporal lobe epilepsy. *J Neurol Neurosurg Psychiatry* **73**, 478-485.

Ehlers, S. Nydén, A., Gillberg, C., Dahlgran-Sandberg, A., Dahlgran, S.-O., Hjelmquist, E. and Odén, A. (1997). Asperger syndrome, autism and attention disorders: a comparative study of the cognitive profile of 120 children. *J Child Psychol Psychiatry* **38**, 207-217.

Engel, J. Jr., Wilson, C, and Lopez-Rodriguez, F. (2002). Limbic connectivity: anatomical substrates of behavioural disturbances in epilepsy. In: Trimble, M.R., and Schmitz, B. (Eds), *The Neuropsychiatry of Epilepsy:* Cambridge University Press, Cambridge, pp. 18-37.

Engel, J.Jr. and Shewmon, D.A. (1991). Impact of the kindling phenomenon on clinical epileptology. In: Morrell, F. (Ed), *Kindling and Synaptic Plasticity: The Legacy of Graham Goddard.* Birkhäuser Boston, Cambridge, Massachusetts, pp. 195-210.

Eschle, D., Siegel, A.M. and Wieser, H.G. (2002) Epilepsy with severe abdominal pain. *Mayo Clin Proc* **77**, 1358-1360.

Fein, D., Pennington, B. and Waterhouse, L. (1987). Implications of social deficits in autism for neurological dysfunction. In: Schopler, E. and Mesibov, G.B. (Eds), *Neurobiological Issues in Autism,* Wiley-Liss, New York, pp. 127-144.

Feindel, W. and Penfield, W. (1954). Localisation of discharge in temporal lobe automatism. *Arch Neurol Psych* **72**, 605-630.

File, S.E., Gonzalez, L.E. and Gallant, R. (1998). Role of the basolateral nucleus of the amygdala in the formation of a phobia. *Neuropsychopharmacology,* **19**, 397-405.

Fine, S.E. (2000). The amygdala: anxiety and benzodiazepines. In: Aggleton, J.P. (Ed), *The Amygdala – A Functional Analysis.* Oxford University Press, Oxford, pp. 195-212.

Fletcher, P.C., Happé, F., Frith ,U., Baker, S.C., Dolan, R.J., Frackowiak, R.S. *et al.* (1995). Other minds in the brain: a functional imaging study of 'theory of mind' in story comprehension. *Cognition,* **57**, 109-128.

Fotheringham, J.B. (1991). Autism and its primary psychosocial and neurological deficit. *Can J Psychiatry* **36**, 686-692.

Frith, U. (1989). Autism and 'theory of mind'. In: Gillberg, Ch. (Ed), *Diagnosis and Treatment of Autism.* New York. Plenum Press, pp. 33-52.

Fuster, J. M. (1997). Human Neuropsychology – Prefrontal Disorders, Prefrontal Sydromes. In: Fuster, J.M. (Ed), *The Prefrontal Cortex. Anatomy, Physiology, and Neuropsychology of the Frontal Lobe* 3rd edn. Lippincott-Raven, Philadelphia, pp. 150-184.

Gallagher, M. (2000). The amygdala and associative learning. In: J.P. Aggleton (Ed.). *The Amygdala - A Functional Analysis* Oxford University Press, Oxford pp. 311-329.

Gallagher H.L., Happé F., Brunswick N., Fletcher P.C., Frith U. and Frith C.D. (2000). Reading the mind in cartoons and stories: an fMRI study of 'theory of mind' in verbal and nonverbal tasks. *Neuropsychology* **38**, 11-21.

George, M.S., Costa, D.C., Kouris, K., Ring, H.A. and Ell, P.J. (1992). Cerebral blood flow in adults with infantile autism. *J Nerv Ment Dis* **180**, 413-417.

Gidd, J.N., Vaituzis, A.C., Hamburger, S.D., Lange, D., Rajapakse, J.C., Kaysan, D., Vauss, Y.C., Rapoport, J.L. *et al.* (1996). Quantitative MRI of the Temporal Lobes, amygdala and hippocampus in normal human development: ages 4-18. *J Comp Neurol* **366**, 223-230.

Gillberg, C. (1983). Autistic children's hand preferences: results from an epidemiological study of infantile autism. *Psychiatry Res* **10**, 21-30.

Gillberg, C. (1991). Clinical and Neurobiological aspects of Asperger Syndrome in six family studies. In: Frith, U. (Ed), *Autism and Asperger Syndrome*. Cambridge University Press, Cambridge, pp. 122-146.

Gillberg , C. (2000a). Asperger Syndrome. In: Gillberg, C, and Coleman, M. (Eds), *The Biology of Autistic Syndromes. 3rd edn* MacKeith Press, London, pp. 39-52.

Gillberg, C. (2000b). The Neurology of Autism (review) In: Gillberg, C, and Coleman, M. (Eds), *The Biology of Autistic Syndromes.* MacKeith Press. London, pp. 291-309.

Gillberg, C. and Coleman, M. (2000). Epilepsy and Electrophysiology. In: Gillberg C. and Coleman M. (Eds), *The Biology of Autistic Syndromes.* MacKeith Press, London, pp. 185-196.

Gillberg, I.C. and Gillberg, C. (1989). Asperger Syndrome – some epidemiological considerations: a research note. *J Child Psychol Psychiatry* **33**, 531-542.

Gillberg, Ch., Gillberg, C., Råstam, M. and Wentz, E. (2001). The Asperger Syndrome (and high-functioning autism) Diagnostic Interview (ASDI): a preliminary study of a new structured clinical interview. *Autism* **5**, 57-66.

Gillberg, C. and Ehlers, S. (1998). High-Functioning People with Autism and Asperger Syndrome: A Literature Review. In: Schopler, E., Mesibov, G., and Kunce, L. (Eds), *Asperger Syndrome or High Functioning Autism? J Aut Dev Dis, Special Issue.* Plenum Press, New York, pp. 79-106.

Gloor, P. (1997). *The Temporal Lobe and the Limbic System.* Oxford University Press, New York.

Goddard, G.V., McIntyre, D.C. and Leech, C.K. (1969). A permanent change in brain function resulting from daily electrical stimulation. *Exp Neurol* **25**, 295-330.

Gonzalez, L.E., Andrews, N. and File, S.E. (1996). 5-HT[1A] and benzodiazepine receptors in the basolateral amygdala modulate anxiety in the social interaction test, but not in the elevated plus maze. *Brain Res* **732**, 145-153.

Gustafsson, L. (1997). Inadequate cortical feature maps: a neural circuit theory of autism. *Biol Psychiatry* **42**, 1138-1147.

Halgren, E., Walter, R.D., Cherlow, D.G. and Crandall, P.H. (1978). Mental phenomena evoked by electrical stimulation of the human hippocampal formation and amygdala. *Brain* **101**, 83-117.

Hare, R.D. and Quinn, M.J. (1971). Psychopathy and autonomic conditioning. *J Abnorm Psychol* **77**, 223-235.

Heaton, P., Germelin, B. and Pring, L. (1999). Can children with autistic spectrum disorders perceive affect in music: An experimental investigation. *Psychol Mec* **29**, 1405-1410.

Heimer, L., Alheid, G.F., de Olmos, J.S., Groenewegen, H.J., Haber, S.N., Harlan, R.E. and Zahm, D.S., (1997). The accumbens: beyond the core-shell dichotomy. *J Neuropsychiatry Clin Neurosci* **9**, 354-381.

Jarrold, C. and Russell, J. (1997). Counting abilities in autism: possible implications for central coherence theory. *J Autism Dev Disord* **27**, 25-37.

Jolliffe, T. and Baron-Cohen, S. (1997). Are people with autism and Asperger Syndrome faster than normal on the Embedded Figures Test? *J Child Psychol Psychiatry* **38**, 527-534.

Kalynchuk, L.E., Pinel, J.P. and Treit, D. (1999). Characterization of the defensive nature of kindling-induced emotionality. *Behav Neurosci* **113**, 766.

Kanner, L. (1943). Autistic disturbances of affective contact. *Nervous Child* **2**, 217-250.

Kawashima, R., Sugiura, M., Kato, T., Nakamura, A., Hatano, K., Ito, K., *et al* (1999). The human amygdala plays an important role in gaze monitoring: a PET study. *Brain* **122**, 779-783.

Kemper, T.L. and Bauman, M. (1998). Neuropathology of infantile autism. *J Neuropathol Exp Neurol* **57**, 645-652.

Kling, A., Lancaster, J. and Bentone, J. (1972). Amygdalectomy in the free ranging vervet. *J Psychiatr Res* **7**, 191-199.

Kling, A. and Brothers, L. (1992). The amygdala and social behaviour. In: Aggleton, J.P. (Ed), *Neurobiological aspects of emotion, memory and mental dysfunction.* Wiley, New York, pp. 353-377.

Klüver, H. and Bucy, P.C. (1937) 'Psychic blindness' and other symptoms following bilateral temporal lobectomy in rhesus monkeys. *Am J Physiol* **119**, 352-353.

Lamprecht, R. and Dudai, Y. (2000). The amygdala in conditioned taste aversion: it's there, but where? In: Aggleton, J.P. (Ed) *The Amygdala – A Functional Analysis.* Oxford University Press, Oxford, pp. 331-352.

LeDoux, J.E. (1996) *The Emotional Brain.* Simon and Schuster, New York.

LeDoux, J.E. (2000). The amygdala and emotion: a view from fear. In: Aggleton, J.P. (Ed), *The Amygdala.- A Functional Analysis.* Oxford University Press, Oxford, pp. 289-310.

Leekam, S., Libby, S., Wing, L., Gould, J. and Gillberg, C. (2000). Comparison of ICD-10 and Gillberg's Criteria for Asperger Syndrome. *Autism* **4**, 11-28.

Levenston, G.K., Patrick, C.J., Bradley, M.M. and Lang, P.J. (2000). The psychopath as observer: emotion and attention in picture processing. *J Abnorm Psychol* **109**, 373-385.

Lezak, M.D. (1995). Theory and Practice of Neuropsychological Assessment. Basic Concepts. In: Lezak, M.D. (Ed), *Neuropschological Assessment. 3rd edn,,* Oxford University Press, New York, pp. 17-44.

Lichter, D.G. and Cummings, J.L. (2001). *Frontal-Subcortical Circuits in Psychiatric and Neurological Disorders.* The Guildford Press, London.

Lord, C., Rutter, M. and LeCouteur, A. (1994). Autism Diagnostic Interview - Revised: A revised version of a diagnostic interview for caregivers of individuals with possible pervasive developmental disorders. *J Autism Dev Disord* **24**(5), 659-685.

MacLean, P.D. (1952). Some psychiatric implications of physiological studies on the frontotemporal portion of limbic system (visceral brain). *EEG Clin Neurophysiol* **4**, 407-418.

MacLean, P.D. (1992). The Limbic System Concept. In: Trimble, M.R. and Bolwig, T.G. (Eds), *The Temporal Lobes and the Limbic System,* Wrightson Biomedical Publishing, Petersfield, pp. 1-14.

McAlonan, G..M., Daly, E., Kumari ,V., Critchley, H.D., Amelsvoort, Th.v., Sucling, J., Simmons, A., Sigmundsson, Th., Greenwood, K., Russell, A., Schmitz, N., Happé, F., Howlin, P. and Murphy, D.G.M. (2002). Brain anatomy and sensorimotor gating in Asperger's Syndrome. *Brain* **127**, 1594-1606.

McLennan, J.D., Lord, C. and Schopler, E. (1993). Sex differences in higher functioning people with autism. *J Aut Dev Diff* **23**, 217-227.

McNamara, J.O. and Wada, J.A.(1997). Kindling Models In: Engel, J. and Pedley, T.A. (Eds), *Epilepsy: A Comprehensive Textbook.* Lippincott-Raven, Philadelphia, pp. 419-425.

Middleton, F. A. (2001). Revised Neuroanatomy of Frontal-Subcortical Circuits. In: Lichter, D.G. and Cummings, J.L. (Eds), *Frontal-Subcortical Circuits in Psychiatric and Neurological Disorders.* The Guilford Press, New York, pp. 44-58.

Minshew, N.J., Goldstein, G. and Siegel, D.J. (1997). Neuropsychological functioning in autism: profile of a complex information processing disorder. *J Int Neuropsychol Soc* **3**, 303-316.

Morris, J.S., Ohman, A. and Dolan, R.J. (1998). Conscious and unconscious emotional learning in the human amygdala. *Nature* **393**, 467-470.

Morris, J.S., Ohman, A. and Dolan, R.J. (1999). A subcortical pathway to the right amygdala mediating 'unseen' fear. *Proc Natl Acad Sci USA* **96**, 1680-1685.

Muller, J., Corodimas, K.P., Fridel, Z. and LeDoux, J.E. (1997). Functional inactivation of the lateral and basal nuclei of the amygdala by muscimol infusion prevents fear conditioning to an explicit CS and to contextual stimuli. *Behav Neurosci* **111**, 683-691.

Niehoff, D.L. and Kuhar, M.J. (1983). Benzodiazepine receptors: localisation in rat amygdala. *J Neurosci* **3**, 2091-2097.

Nydén, A., Gillberg, C., Hjelmquist, E. and Heimann, M. (1999). Executive function/attention in boys with Asperger syndrome, attention disorders and reading/writing disorder. Autism **3**, 213-228.

Onoe, H., Tsukada, H., Nishiyama, S., Nakanishi, S., Inoue, O. and Langstrom, B. (1996). A subclass of GABAₐ/benzodiazepine receptor exclusively localised in the limbic system. *Neuroreport* **8**, 117-122.

Otsuka, H., Harada, M., Mori, K., Hisaoka, S., Nishitani, H., *et al.* (1999). Brain metabolites in the hippocampal-amygdala region and cerebellum in autism: an 1-H spectroscopy study. *Neuroradiology* **41**, 517-519

Ozonoff, S. and Miller, J.N. (1996). An exploration of right-hemisphere contribution to the pragmatic impairments of autism. *Brain Lang* **52**, 411-434.

Papez, J.W. (1937). A proposed mechanism of emotion. *Arch Neurol Psych* **38**, 725-743.

Penfield, W. and Rasmussen, T (1957). In: Penfield, W. and Rasmussen, T. (Eds), *The Cerebral Cortex of Man.* Macmillan, New York, pp. 77-86.

Pitkänen, A., Tuunanen, J., Kälviäienen, R., Partanen, K. And Salmenperä, T. (1998). Amygdala damage in experimental and human epilepsy. *Epilepsy Res* **328**, 233-253.

Pitkänen, A. (2000). Connectivity of the rat amygdaloid complex. In: Aggleton, J.P. (Ed), *The Amygdala – A Functional Analysis.* Oxford University Press, Oxford, pp. 31-116.

Piven, J., Saliba, K., Bailey, J. and Arndt, S. (1997). An MRI study of autism: the cerebellum revisited. *Neurology* **49**, 546-551.

Piven, J., Bailey, J., Ranson, B.J. and Arndt, S. (1998). No difference in hippocampus volume detected on magnetic resonance imaging in autistic individuals. *J Autism Dev Disord* **28**, 105-110.

Pribram, K.H. and Bagshaw, M. (1953). Further analysis of the temporal lobe syndrome utilising frontotemporal ablations. *J Comp Neurol* **99**, 347-375.

Price, J.L., Russchen, F.T. and Amaral, D.G. (1987). The limbic region. II: The amygdaloid complex. In: Björklund, B., Hokfelt, T. and Swanson, L.W. (Eds), *Handbook of Chemical Neuroanatomy. Vol 5, Integrated Systems of the CNS, Part I.* Elsevier, Amsterdam, pp. 279-388.

Quirk, G.J., Armony, J.L. and LeDoux, J.E. (1997). Fear conditioning enhances different temporal components of tone-evoked spike trains in auditory cortex and lateral amygdala. *Neuron* **19**, 613-624.

Rolls, E.T. (2000). Neurophysiology and functions of the primate amygdala, and the neural basis of emotion. In: Aggleton, J.P. (Ed), *The Amygdala - A Functional Analysis.* Oxford University Press, Oxford, pp. 447-478.

Ross, E.D. (1993). Nonverbal aspects of language. *Neurol Clin* **11**, 9-23.

Rosvold, H.E., Mirsky, A.F. and Pribram, K.H. (1954). Influence of amygdalectomy on social behaviour in monkeys. *J Comp Physiol Psychol* **47**, 173-178.

Rutter, M., Gailey, A., Bolton, P. and Le Couteur, A. (1993). Autism: Syndrome definition and possible genetic mechanisms. In: Plomin, R. and McClearn, G.E. (Eds), *Nature, Nuture, and Psychology.* American Psychological Association, Washington, DC, pp. 269-284.

Schwartzkroin, P.A. and McIntryre, D.C. (1997). Limbic Anatomy and Physiology. In: Engel, J. Jr. and Pedley, T.A. (Eds), *Epilepsy: A Comprehensive Textbook.* Lippincott-Raven, Philadelphia, pp. 323-340.

Scott, S.K., Young, A.W., Calder, A.J., Hellawell, D.J., Aggleton, J.P. and Johnson, M. (1997). Impaired auditory recognition of fear and anger following bilateral amygdala lesions. *Nature* **385**, 254-257.

Shammah-Lagnado, S.J., Alheid, G.G. and Heimer, L. (2001). Striatal and central extended amygdala parts of the interstitial nucleus of the posterior nucleus of the posterior limb of the anterior commissure: evidence from tractotracing techniques in the rat. *J Comp Neurol* **439**, 104-126.

Soderstrom, H., Rastam, M. and Gillberg, Ch. (2002). Temperament and character in adultes with Asperger Syndrome. *Autism* **6**(3), 287-298.

Staufenberg, E.F.A. (1994). Asperger Syndrome and Affective Disorders: A Family History Study of Unipolar Depression, Bipolar Disorder, Schizophrenia, and Schizo-Affective Disorder in First Degree Relatives. MSc Thesis, Victoria University, Manchester, UK.

Stefan, H. (1999). Plasticity and Epilepsy: An Outline of the Problem. In: Stefan, H., Andermann, F., Chauvel, P. and Shorvon, S.D. (Eds), *Advances in Neurology, Vol. 81, Plasticity in Epilepsy: Dynamic Aspects of Brain Function.* Lippincott Williams & Wilkins, Philadelphia, pp 1-6.

Stone, W.L., Ousley, O.Y., Yoder, P.J., Hogan, K.L. and Hepburn, S.L. (1997). Nonverbal communication in two-and three year old children with autism. *J Autism Dev Disord* **27**, 677-696.

Stuss, D.T., Gallup, G.G. and Alexander, M.P. (2002). The frontal lobes are necessary for 'theory of mind'. *Brain* **124**, 124-286.

Thomas, D.M., Drevet, W.C., Whalen, P.J., Eccard, C.H., Dall, R.E., Ryan, N.D., Casey, B.J. *et al.* (2001). Amygdala response to facial expression in children and adults. *Biol Psychiatry* **49**(4), 309-316.

Torrey, E.F., Hersh, S.P. and McCabe, K.D. (1975). Early childhood psychosis and bleeding during pregnancy: a prospective study of gravid children and their offspring. *J Aut Childhood Schiz* **5**, 287-297.

Trimble, M.R. and Schmitz, B. (2002). *The Neuropsychiatry of Epilepsy.* Cambridge University Press, Cambridge.

van Elst, L.T. (2002). Aggression and epilepsy. In: Trimble, M.R. and Schmitz, B. (Eds), *The Neuropsychiatry of Epilepsy.* Cambridge University Press, Cambridge, pp. 81-106.

Vogeley, K., Bussfeld, P., Newen, A., Herrmann, S., Happé, F., Falkai, P. *et al.* (2001). Mind reading: neural mechanisms of theory of mind and self-perspective. *Neuroimage* **14**, 170-181.

Volkmar, F.R., McLennan, J.D., Lord, C. and Schopler, E. (1993a). Sex differences in higher functioning people with autism. *J Autism Dev Disord* **23**, 217-227.

Volkmar, F.R., Szatmari, P. and Sparrow, S.S. (1993b). Sex differences in pervasive developmental disorders. *J Autism Dev Disord* **23**, 759-591.

Webster, M.J., Ungerleider, L.G. and Bachevalier, J. (1991). Connections of inferior temporal areas TE and TEO with medial temporal lobe structures in infant and adult monkeys. *J Neurosci*, **11** (4), 1095-1116.

Wilensky, A.E., Schafe, G.E. and LeDoux, J.E. (2000). The amygdala modulates memory consolidation of fear-motivated inhibitory avoidance learning but not classical fear conditioning. *J Neurosci* **20**, 7059-7066.

Wilson, F.A.W., Richens, I.P. and Brown, M.W. (1990). Hippocampus and medial temporal cortex: neuronal responses related to behavioural responses during the performance of memory tasks by primates. *Behav Brain Res* **40**, 7-28.

Wing, L. and Gould, J. (1979). Severe impairments of social interaction and associated abnormalities in children: epidemiology and classification. *J Autism Dev Disord* **9**, 11-29.

Young, M.P., Scannell, J.W., Burns, G.A.P.C. and Blakemore, C. (1994). Analysis of connectivity: neural systems in the cerebral cortex. *Rev Neurosci* **5**, 227-249.

Zald, D.H. and Pardo, J.V. (1997). Emotion, olfaction, and the human amygdala: amygdala activation during aversive olfactory stimulation. *Proc Nat Acad Sci USA* **94**, 4119-4124.

Zilbovicius, M., Garreau, B., Samson, Y., Remy, P., Barthelemy, C., Syrot, A. and Lelord, G. (1995). Delayed maturation of the frontal cortex in childhood. *Am J Psychiatry*, 152-252.

7

The EEG and Learning Disability

FRANK M.C. BESAG

Bedfordshire and Luton Community NHS Trust,
University of Luton, Luton, UK
and Centre for Epilepsy, Maudsley Hospital, London, UK

INTRODUCTION

EEG abnormalities may be associated with cognitive problems in a number of different ways. First, it is important to distinguish between the EEG abnormalities that cause cognitive problems and those that are associated with but do not cause the cognitive difficulties. These two situations are illustrated in Figure 1. The first of these two situations will be discussed in detail. The second situation commonly arises when there is some underlying structural or functional brain problem that leads to both learning disability and also, independently, to EEG changes. For example, it is common for individuals who have severe learning disability to have a constant non-specific slow-wave abnormality in the EEG. This EEG abnormality is not treatable and would not generally be considered to be the cause of the learning disability. Both the learning disability and the EEG abnormality are the consequence of the underlying brain problem. With regard to cognitive problems that do arise from EEG abnormalities, these may be divided into ictal and post-ictal. The question of inter-ictal discharges causing cognitive problems raises some interesting semantic questions about the definition of a seizure, which will be discussed further in the section on transitory cognitive impairment (TCI).

The issue of recognising treatable, reversible cognitive impairment resulting from epilepsy is of major importance. In this context it may be helpful to discuss the concepts of permanent learning disability on the one hand and state-dependent learning disability on the other. These concepts have been presented elsewhere (Besag, 2001). As already stated, permanent learning disability may arise independently from the brain damage or

Figure 1

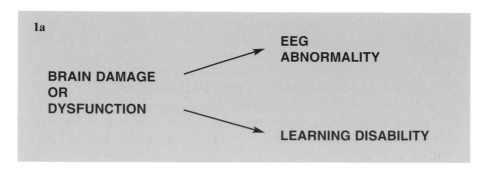

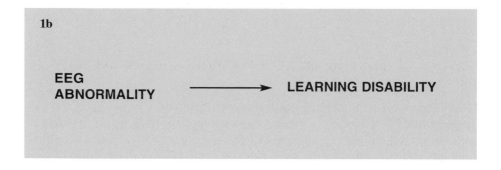

Table 1. A classification of the causes of state-dependent learning disability.

1.	**Ictal**
(i)	Frequent spike-wave discharges associated with absence seizures (Non-convulsive status epilepticus)
(ii)	Complex partial status epilepticus
(iii)	Focal discharges (a) Transitory cognitive impairment (TCI) (b) Frequent localised discharges (c) Frequent hemispheric discharges
2.	**Post-ictal**
(i)	EEG slowing from frequent daytime seizures
(ii)	EEG slowing from frequent night-time seizures
(iii)	ESES
(iv)	Other epileptiform discharges

dysfunction that caused the epilepsy to develop. Alternatively, permanent brain damage and consequently permanent learning disability may result from the epilepsy itself. The familiar situation is the person who has had an episode of prolonged status epilepticus that has caused both permanent brain damage and, as a result, permanent learning disability. This epilepsy-associated cognitive impairment must be distinguished from the types of state-dependent cognitive impairment that can result from epilepsy. These are listed in Table 1. The different categories in this Table will be discussed in detail. However, first a number of the childhood syndromes associated with learning disability will be described. Several of these will then be related to the categories in Table 1.

AN OVERVIEW OF EPILEPSY SYNDROMES OF CHILDHOOD ASSOCIATED WITH LEARNING DISABILITY AND EEG ABNORMALITIES.

Ohtahara syndrome: early-infantile epileptic encephalopathy with suppression-bursts

This syndrome is characterised by onset within the first few months of life, of frequent tonic seizures and repeated suppression-burst patterns in the EEG, during both waking and sleeping states (Ohtahara et al., 1992). The outcome is poor. Many of the infants with this syndrome die early. Those who survive are likely to have the severe learning disability and refractory seizures. Ohtahara syndrome may evolve into the West syndrome and sometimes into the Lennox-Gastaut syndrome. An underlying pathology such as porencephaly, Aicardi syndrome or a cortical malformation is commonly found. Of 15 cases reported in the review of Ohtahara et al. (1992), seven died and all 15 had severe learning disability. In some of the surviving cases the suppression-burst pattern on the EEG was replaced by hypsarrhythmia in later infancy.

The Ohtahara syndrome is probably an example of the situation illustrated in Figure 1a, namely both the epilepsy and learning disability arising from an underlying brain pathology. Because these infants are often very resistant to anti-epileptic treatment it is difficult to determine whether effective treatment that improves the EEG would also improve cognition. Even if both the EEG changes and the poor cognition are the result of underlying pathology, improving the brain function by suppressing the EEG abnormality might result in some limited improvement in cognition. With the increasing range of anti-epileptic drugs becoming available, it might be possible to discover the answer to these questions.

West syndrome

West Syndrome was originally described by Dr West in his own son (West, 1841). It is characterised by infantile spasms, learning disability and hypsarrhythmia on the EEG. The onset is most commonly between around 4 and 7 months. Flexion spasms are reported in 68%. The flexion spasms are often referred to as 'salaam spasms', because they resemble the salaam, a low bow of obeisance. Extensor, lightning and nodding spasms also occur. The spasms tend to occur in episodes. 30-100 spasms may occur in one episode. Several episodes may occur per day. There is sometimes an ictal or post-ictal cry. Cases are divided into symptomatic, in which there is a clear underlying cause and cryptogenic, in which no definite causal pathology can be identified. West syndrome has previously been considered to have a poor prognosis, both in terms of intellectual outcome and with regard to subsequent seizure control. However, it seems that the advent of new and effective anti-epileptic treatment may be changing the situation – see section on generalised discharges. West syndrome may evolve into the Lennox-Gastaut syndrome as the child grows older.

Dravet syndrome: severe myoclonic epilepsy in infancy.

Dravet syndrome is characterised by seizure onset in the first year of life, usually with febrile convulsions or generalised clonic seizures, followed by myoclonic and/or partial/typical absence seizures between 2 and 3 years of age (Dravet et al., 1992). There is delayed development from the second year and unsteadiness is generally seen. Initially the EEG does not usually show paroxysmal abnormalities but in the second year of life inter-ictal generalised spike-wave complexes and/or generalised polyspike-wave discharges are present. This is one of the childhood epilepsies that has generally been considered to be very resistant to treatment. However, Nieto-Barrera et al. (2000) demonstrated a good response to topiramate in a group of 18 patients, in whom over half had a reduction in seizure frequency by more than 50%. Three became free of seizures. The best response was in atypical absence seizures. Cognitive testing and serial EEG results were not reported in this series. It will be important to collect such data in future series. It seems highly likely that children with the Dravet Syndrome who respond well to treatment with the new anti-epileptic drugs available will have a much better cognitive outcome than was reported in the past for children with this syndrome.

Lennox-Gastaut Syndrome.

The Lennox-Gastaut syndrome is characterised by axial tonic seizures, atypical absence seizures, atonic/myoclonic seizures, slow spike-wave discharges, around two per second, in the EEG and fast rhythmic bursts of 10 per second frequency during sleep (Gastaut *et al.*, 1966). The onset is usually under eight years of age, with a peak at 3-5 years. Cognitive development is particularly poor. In the past, before the newer anti-epileptic drugs became available, 60-80% continued to have seizures, despite treatment. The prognosis now appears to be better but longer-term analyses of large series will need to be performed before reliable up-to-date figures for seizure and cognitive outcome can be provided.

A CLASSIFICATION OF THE CAUSES OF STATE-DEPENDENT LEARNING DISABILITY

A suggested classification of the causes of state-dependent learning disability is shown in Table 1. These causes will be discussed in turn.

1. ICTAL

(i)   Frequent generalised discharges

(a) Absence seizures and non-convulsive status epilepticus

The relatively infrequent absence seizures that occur in many children with classical absence epilepsy do not appear to have any effect on cognitive outcome. It is interesting to note that they may put the child at risk from other causes. For example, the accident rate in children with absence seizures is remarkably high. If the absence seizures occur in social situations the child may lose confidence and this may affect schooling. They can also have poor classroom performance because the child is briefly unaware of what the teacher or others are saying during the absence seizure. It appears the children who have infrequent absence seizures cope with this situation quite well. However, if the absence seizures are very frequent they may impinge in a significant way on learning.

Frequent absence seizures may also lead to fragmented thought processes. Some people with the frequent absence seizures have very disjointed expressive language which might even be mistaken for the 'word salad' of schizophrenia. The EEG should be diagnostic in this situation. If an EEG performed at the time when the language appears disjointed reveals frequent spike-wave discharges, then it is likely that the discharges are causing the problem.

Inattention may be caused by frequent absence seizures and this state may mimic some of the features of attention deficit hyperactivity disorder. The child may appear generally disorganised and exhibit motor overactivity along with the inattention. The appropriate treatment in such cases is suitable anti-epileptic medication, not the stimulant medication that would be used for classical attention deficit hyperactivity disorder.

It is important to emphasise the fact that anti-epileptic treatment, in some cases, may be unsuccessful in controlling the overt seizures while being highly

Figure 2a. Case A: Overt seizures (top) and spike and wave events (bottom).

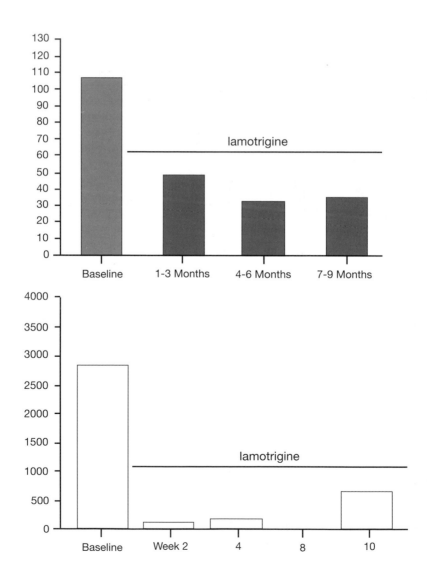

effective in controlling the absence seizures (or vice versa). Most clinicians assess the success or failure of anti-epileptic medication by a reduction in the overt seizures. This may lead to incorrect management decisions. The situation is well illustrated by two cases from the author's experience. In the first

Figure 2b. Case B: Overt seizures (top) and spike and wave events (bottom).

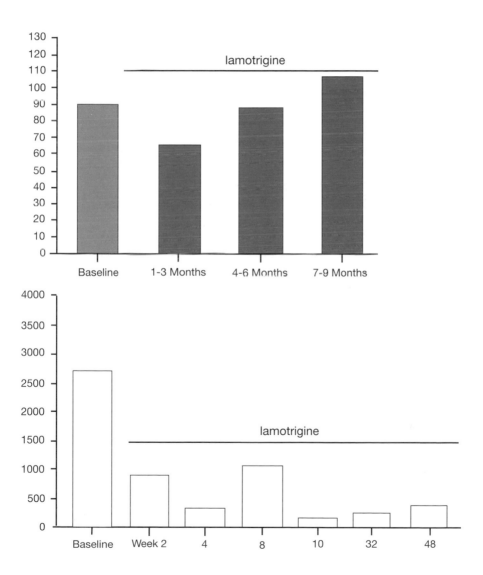

case, illustrated in Figure 2a, both the overt seizures and the spike-wave discharges were reduced by introducing lamotrigine. In the second case, illustrated in Figure 2b, the overt seizures were unaffected by the lamotrigine but the spike-wave discharges were reduced by more than 2000 per day, resulting in great clinical benefit to the patient, who became alert and in control of his life again. If the lamotrigine had been stopped in the second case, on the basis that there had been no reduction in overt seizures, the frequent spike-wave discharges would almost certainly have returned and the patient would have been greatly disabled as a result.

Of course, the best situation would be to control both the overt seizures and the subtle seizures completely but it would be a serious mistake to miss the opportunity of controlling the handicapping subtle seizures by failing to assess the situation properly. Ideally, such patients should have serial prolonged EEG monitoring to determine that the anti-epileptic medication is continuing to be effective in controlling the spike-wave episodes. The current author's group developed an automatic spike-wave monitor to facilitate the follow-up of these patients (Besag *et al.*, 1989). The examples just given illustrate how valuable such EEG monitoring can be. Sometimes follow-up monitoring reveals that the spike-wave episodes have returned after a period of control. Figure 3 illustrates this situation. In this case, allowance had not been made for the fact that the child had grown and gained in weight. When the dose of the anti-epileptic medication was increased, almost complete

Figure 3. Lamotrigine: number of spike-wave events

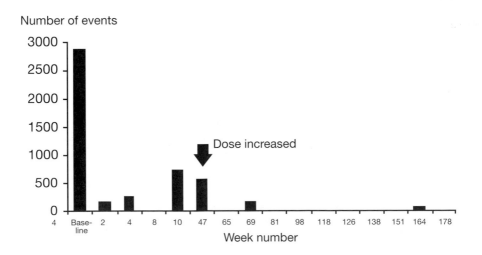

control of the spike-wave episodes was achieved and this was maintained over years of subsequent follow-up.

The extreme example of the way in which frequent generalised spike-wave discharges can impair cognition is absence non-convulsive status epilepticus (Cascino, 1993; Stores *et al.*, 1995). In this condition the spike-wave discharges occur so frequently that the person cannot recover function between them. The EEG confirms the diagnosis, showing very frequent generalised spike-wave discharges. Sometimes the whole record is occupied by these discharges. The range of clinical manifestations of non-convulsive status epilepticus is surprisingly broad. Some children are able to speak and appear to be interacting at a reasonable level, although they may seem quieter than usual. Other children enter a 'zombie-like' state in which they are unable to speak, walk or even support their own weight. The degree of abnormality on the EEG does not seem to correlate with the severity of the clinical manifestations. For example, even if the EEG shows continuous spike-wave discharges, the person may nevertheless be able to walk, respond to a question by making a sound and look around, apparently taking an interest in their surroundings. On the other hand, intermittent spike-wave discharges may be accompanied by the 'zombie-like' state described earlier. Because the manifestations of non-convulsive status epilepticus vary so widely, less obvious cases may be missed. Unfortunately, sometimes even the more obvious cases are missed because no-one has thought of non-convulsive status epilepticus as being a possible diagnosis for that particular patient. If there is any suspicion of this condition, an urgent EEG should be performed. It is very important to note that the EEG must be carried out while the person is in the altered state. If the individual has returned to normal by the time the EEG is performed, no useful information may be gained.

(b) West syndrome

In West syndrome (Renier, 2000; West, 1841), the generalised discharges are seen as hypsarrhythmia, a grossly abnormal, highly disorganised pattern of high-voltage slow waves and spikes on the EEG. It is interesting to note that children who develop infantile spasms typically lose skills and subsequently develop poorly. The condition was previously considered to be difficult to treat, although some cases responded to ACTH or steroids. However, in recent years, vigabatrin has been shown to be highly effective, especially if the cause of the West Syndrome is tuberous sclerosis.

There now seems to be good evidence to suggest that suppression of the seizures and the hypsarrhythmia may be associated with improvement in cognitive function. This provides another example in which early effective treatment may be important for the cognitive development of the child. If the seizures are secondary to focal pathology, surgical treatment may be feasible as discussed later in this chapter. Jambaqué *et al.* (2000) demonstrated that children with infantile spasms who were successfully treated with vigabatrin showed a significant increase in mental score and an improvement in behaviour, although most of them continued to have partial seizures. De Menezes and Rho (2002) have reported that, in children whose spasms persisted beyond the first year of life, a disorganised EEG background and continuing hypsarrhythmia were associated with a poor developmental outcome. This again supports the concept that abolishing the abnormal EEG discharges might result in a better cognitive prognosis, although it could be argued that the more abnormal EEG is a consequence rather than a cause of the ongoing brain problem.

The evidence from prompt medical and (see later) surgical treatment of West Syndrome suggests strongly that control of the underlying EEG disturbance can be associated with improvements in cognition. These treatments may also prevent permanent deterioration in cognitive ability, in at least some cases.

(c) Lennox-Gastaut syndrome

In the Lennox-Gastaut syndrome, the seizures have, in the past, been considered as being very refractory to treatment. However, good responses have been seen with some of the new antiepileptic drugs, notably lamotrigine (Motte *et al.*, 1997). Many children with the Lennox-Gastaut syndrome probably have hundreds of atypical absence seizures daily. Control of these seizures is accompanied by clear improvement in alertness and performance, but there is a lack of good follow-up studies with sequential cognitive testing and EEG monitoring.

(ii) Complex Partial Seizure Status Epilepticus

There are several reports of prolonged complex partial seizure status epilepticus (Cascino, 1993). This may be much more difficult to diagnose because the EEG abnormality is not so obvious. However, if it is suspected, then an urgent EEG is again an appropriate investigation. There is some evidence that prolonged localised seizure activity may cause brain damage, implying the possibility that it might cause specific cognitive impairment of a permanent nature.

(iii) Frequent Focal Discharges

(a) Transitory Cognitive Impairment (TCI)

The phenomenon of transitory cognitive impairment (TCI) has been reviewed by Binnie and colleagues, (Aarts *et al.*, 1984; Binnie *et al.*, 1990; Binnie and

Marston, 1992) who have carried out a number of studies in this area. The underlying concept of transitory cognitive impairment is that epileptiform discharges that are not manifested as seizures detected by simple observation may nevertheless impair cognitive function. Although the cognitive impairment itself may be transitory, the person experiencing this phenomenon may find the situation frustrating and may lose confidence, with the result that schooling is affected.

Marston et al. (1993) found that anti-epileptic drug treatment of children with transitory cognitive impairment was associated with an improvement in the psychosocial function. However, this study was confounded by the fact that the medication not only reduced epileptiform discharges but also reduced the frequency of the obvious seizures. Ronen et al. (2000) failed to demonstrate any improvement in learning in eight children, aged 6-12 years who had epileptiform discharges and were treated with sodium valproate. They found the treatment with valproate was associated with reduced ability rather than improvement on verbal memory tasks. There were also increased delays on intentional tasks and increased parental reports of internalising problems. However, this study was small and the sample was heterogeneous. Furthermore, the paroxysmal EEG discharges improved in only four of the eight children. In three children the number of discharges was similar on treatment and in the remaining child the number of discharges increased.

A more recent study by Pressler et al. (submitted for publication – personal communication) confirmed that reducing epileptiform discharges with lamotrigine treatment improved behaviour in children. Their study is interesting because the children who were treated with lamotrigine but did not have a reduction in epileptiform discharges showed no improvement in behaviour whereas those who did show a reduction in the epileptiform discharges were found to have improved in terms of behaviour. This would appear to indicate that the improvement was not a direct effect of the lamotrigine itself because it occurred only in those showing a reduction in the epileptiform discharges.

As indicated earlier, success in school may be affected by a number of factors. If the child lacks confidence or exhibits behavioural problems, even if there is no demonstrable deficit on formal cognitive testing, schooling and academic progress may be affected adversely.

The frequent localised discharges associated with the so-called benign epilepsy with centrotemporal spikes (BECTS) or Rolandic epilepsy are of particular interest. In the past it was stated that this syndrome was not associated with any cognitive problems. However, Binnie et al. (1992) have pointed out that some of these children do have cognitive problems in school. It was suggested that the frequent focal discharges could result in specific cognitive impairment. Saint-Martin et al. (2001) have also stated that, although children with Rolandic epilepsy generally have normal global intellectual ability and a good long-term prognosis, some have transient neuropsychological deficits.

They have reported that analysis of cognitive and neurophysiological correlations showed a significant correlation between the epileptic focus localisation and the specific cognitive dysfunction. If this is the case, then there is a stronger argument for treating these children with anti-epileptic medication, provided the positive effects on cognition through reducing the discharges are greater than any negative effects of the anti-epileptic medication itself.

It is also interesting to note that there seems to be some overlap between this syndrome and the Landau-Kleffner syndrome, which is discussed in a later section. It has been suggested that while many children with BECTS have no obvious cognitive problems, some may develop the Landau-Kleffner syndrome. Perhaps there is a spectrum of conditions from the truly benign partial seizures with centrotemporal spikes through to children who have centrotemporal spikes but also have electrical status epilepticus of slow-wave sleep. The importance of this is that clinicians should be aware of the possibility of cognitive loss in children who have the EEG pattern typical of benign partial seizures. Specific enquiry should always be made about loss of skills in such children. If there is clear loss of skills then overnight EEG monitoring is justifiable. If this reveals spike-wave discharges then treatment to suppress the discharges is justifiable on the basis that this may be accompanied by a return in cognitive skills (see later section on ESES).

(b) Frequent Localised Discharges

There is a lack of good studies on the effect of frequent localised epileptiform discharges which are not sufficient to cause non-convulsive status epilepticus but are sufficient to cause non-transitory impairment. Frequent fontal discharges can result in highly disinhibited behaviour which may affect the child's performance both in the classroom and in social situations. Dominant temporal discharges may affect verbal abilities, as shown by a number of studies, including those of Stores and co-workers (Stores and Hart, 1975). When the source of frequent dominant temporal epileptiform discharges is removed, speech may improve in some cases.

Westerveld et al. (2000) reported on the cognitive outcome of temporal lobectomy in 82 patients aged 6-17 years. It is interesting to note that only 9% (7 patients: 3 left, 4 right) improved in verbal IQ after surgery and 16% (13 patients: 10 left, 3 right) improved in performance IQ after the surgery. The effect of temporal lobectomy was recently reviewed by the current author (Besag, 2002). It was pointed out that a major omission from the current literature is any adequate discussion of the role of the pre-operative EEG. Did the children who improved have abnormal EEGs before the surgery with frequent epileptiform discharges that were abolished by the surgery? In those who did not improve in cognitive terms, was there any change in the EEG? It tends to be assumed that any decline in cognitive performance after a temporal lobectomy is the result of removal of brain tissue but, in some cases, it is possible that the decline may be partly related to a deterioration in the EEG with an increase in epileptiform discharges. This may particularly be the case if antiepileptic medication is reduced on the basis that obvious seizures are no longer occurring. If, for example, there is a suspicion that some cognitive abilities declined as the medication was reduced, even though the seizures appeared no worse, EEG monitoring would be strongly advisable. If frequent EEG discharges were found then re-institution of appropriate anti-epileptic medication would be appropriate, followed by careful reassessment of both the EEG and the cognitive abilities.

The particularly interesting situation in which epileptiform discharges of focal onset may be accompanied by gross developmental problems is that of babies with infantile spasms in whom focal metabolic abnormalities can be demonstrated by positron emission tomography (PET). Chugani and co-workers have demonstrated that cognitive outcome was remarkably good in some of the patients undergoing surgery to remove the source of the epileptiform discharges (Chugani et al., 1993; Chugani, 1995).

(c) Frequent Hemispheric Discharges

The extreme example of frequent localised discharges is the individual who has an abnormal hemisphere which is a continuous source of epileptiform discharges. A number of pathological conditions can cause this situation. These include hemimegalencephaly, Rasmussen's encephalitis and congenital malformations such as porencephalic cysts. Hemispherectomy, involving either the removal or disconnection of the cerebral cortex on the entire affected side, abolishes the discharges and increases learning in at least some cases. For example, Oxbury et al. (1995) reported an increase in IQ on follow-up after hemispherectomy, with an average of 15 points gain at 5 years.

Several reviews have confirmed the good outcome of hemispherectomy in carefully selected children (Goodman, 1986; Lindsay et al., 1987; Knight and Oxbury, 2000; Oxbury et al., 1995).

2. POST-ICTAL

(i) EEG slowing from frequent daytime seizures

It could be argued that post-ictal slowing is an EEG change that accompanies the temporary cognitive after-effects of the preceding seizure, rather than the EEG slowing *causing* the lowering of the cognitive abilities. In any case, the immediate post-ictal effects of seizures are so obvious that a discussion of them in this context might appear trivial. In practice, however, post-ictal slowing both of the EEG and of cognitive abilities can easily be missed in some circumstances. The following example from the current author's experience illustrates this important situation well (Besag, 1994).

A 16-year-old lad had a single seizure at 5 years and recurrent seizures from 7 years. He then had 20 to 30 bouts of status epilepticus lasting at least 20 minutes. He subsequently had several seizures a day. He sat rocking in his chair, disorientated in time and space, being unable to string words together into a sentence. His mental state was reminiscent of that of an elderly person with dementia. He wandered at night, not knowing where he was. The teaching staff in the special centre in which he had been placed stated that he should not have been accepted because he could not benefit from the educational programmes; his place should have been offered to a child who could have benefited from the placement. The introduction of a second-line antiepileptic drug, which had not previously been tried, transformed him. The seizures were completely controlled and he began reading again. He was able to carry out sensible conversations, to take an active part in domestic chores and to socialise with his peers. The staff in the special centre then remarked on how well he was responding to their educational programmes and how good it was that he was placed in their centre, where he could benefit so much.

This was a dramatic case of state-dependent post-ictal intellectual impairment in someone who was having such frequent seizures that he did not have time to recover from one seizure before the next occurred. When he emerged from this constant post-ictal state, he was able to function at a much higher cognitive level and could benefit from the education available to him. His parents and carers had previously thought that his course would be one of relentless deterioration. The important point is that frequent daytime seizures may lead to a constant post-ictal state that may be mistaken for permanent cognitive impairment, when it is actually state-dependent, treatable, reversible cognitive impairment.

(ii)   EEG slowing from frequent nocturnal seizures

A careful review of overnight video-EEG recordings carried out by the author's group at a specialist centre revealed 15 cases of unsuspected and unobserved nocturnal seizures. Most of these young people were supervised by awake night staff. Despite this, the seizures were missed before the video telemetry was performed. Many of the seizures were relatively brief and some consisted merely of stiffening for a few seconds, accompanied by unequivocal epileptic activity on the EEG. It is quite understandable that the seizures might easily have been missed if it were not for the simultaneous EEG recording. In one of the teenagers monitored in this way, over 200 seizures were recorded in a single night. In some of the subjects, it was quite clear that several of the nocturnal seizures were followed by wakening. This implies that, on the following day, the subject would not only have the post-ictal effects of the seizures themselves but would also have had to contend with the consequences of a very broken night's sleep. If an individual with a history of epilepsy seems to be performing poorly during the daytime, especially if the performance is variable, and perhaps most especially if the performance is particularly bad in the mornings, then the possibility of frequent unobserved nocturnal seizures must be considered. Simple observation, even by an observer who is awake all night, does not necessarily reveal the seizures. Video telemetry is a much more sensitive and reliable way of detecting frequent nocturnal seizures. Effective treatment of the nocturnal seizures gives the person the best opportunity of functioning to their full cognitive ability during the daytime. Post-ictal slow waves on the daytime EEG may provide a clue to seizures having occurred the night before. Although this finding is non-specific, it might raise the suspicion of the doctor carrying out the assessment, especially if daytime performance is variable.

(iii) Electrical status epilepticus of slow-wave sleep (ESES)

Electrical status epilepticus of slow-wave sleep (ESES) provides one of the most striking examples of a link between EEG changes and cognitive problems, notably the Landau-Kleffner syndrome of acquired epileptic aphasia. The term ESES has been debated. The term 'continuous spikes and waves during slow sleep' (CSWS) was adopted by the International League Against Epilepsy Commission on Classification and Terminology. This syndrome is associated with the name of Tassinari, who has carried out classical work in the field. Good reviews have been published by Tassinari *et al.* (2000) and Beaumanoir (1992). The definition of 'Epilepsy with CSWS' provided by the Commission on Classification is as follows.

'Epilepsy with continuous spike-waves during slow sleep results from the association of various seizure types, partial or generalized, occurring during sleep, and atypical absences when awake. Tonic seizures do not occur. The characteristic EEG pattern consists of continuous diffuse spike-waves during slow wave sleep, which is noted after onset of seizures. Duration varies from months to years. Despite the usually benign evolution of seizures, prognosis is guarded, because of the appearance of neuropsychological disorders.'

However, it is important to point out that CSWS may occur in the absence of any obvious seizures and that, even without seizures, the EEG abnormality may be associated with serious cognitive deterioration. For example, it has been suggested that between one quarter and one third of the children with the Landau-Kleffner syndrome do not have obvious seizures, but these children have the very serious cognitive impairment of auditory agnosia. Tassinari (Tassinari, *et al.*, 2000) has stated that encephalopathy with ESES (or ESES syndrome) may be defined as an age-related and self-limited disorder of unknown aetiology characterised by the following features:

1. neuropsychological impairment, in the form of global or selective regression of cognitive functions;

2. motor impairment in the form of ataxia, dyspraxia, dystonia or unilateral deficit;

3. epilepsy, with focal and apparently generalised seizures (unilateral or bilateral clonic seizures, tonic-clonic seizures, absences, partial motor seizures, complex partial seizures or epileptic falls); tonic seizures never occur;

4. typical EEG findings, with ESES pattern occurring during at least 85% of slow sleep and persisting on three or more records over a period of at least one month.

ESES is probably quite rare in childhood epilepsy. Tassinari and colleagues (Tassinari *et al.*, 2000), in their review, quote various series suggesting that it accounts for 0.2-0.5% of all childhood epilepsies, but it should be noted that these were selected populations. The prevalence in childhood epilepsy in the general population is probably even lower.

Although the Landau-Kleffner Syndrome of acquired epileptic aphasia is the classical example of cognitive deterioration in association with ESES, as already stated, a variety of other neuropsychological deficits may occur. One of the earliest reports of children with cognitive deficits in association with frequent spike-wave complexes in slow sleep was that of Patry *et al.* (1971), who reported six children, five of whom had epilepsy and all of whom had learning disability. Two of the six had not acquired speech. However, the clinical condition of acquired epileptic aphasia had been described much earlier by Landau and Kleffner in 1957 (Landau and Kleffner, 1957). The typical situation is that a child, after normal early development, develops auditory agnosia and consequently loses the ability to understand speech. The ability to interpret environmental sounds such as bird song may also be lost. Because these children cannot understand their own speech they may become mute.

Referring to the broader category of ESES, not necessarily specifically associated with acquired aphasia, Tassinari has commented that the majority of patients have normal psychological and motor functions before the onset of ESES. Some have abnormal development before the ESES is first recorded. He has stated that all cases exhibit further decrease in cognitive function during the phase in which ESES occurs. The loss of cognitive function may be severe. Cognitive disturbances may include various patterns of decrease in language ability, impairment of global IQ, temporo-spatial disorientation, behavioural changes, including reduced attention span, hyperkinesis, aggressiveness, difficulty in contact and, rarely, psychotic states.

Although the ESES seems to resolve in all cases and the seizures are also said to have a benign prognosis, the outcome in terms of permanent cognitive deficits is very variable. The argument for early treatment to suppress the ESES seems to be gaining strength. For example, Robinson *et al.* (2001) examined the outcome of 18 children with the Landau-Kleffner Syndrome and found that no child with ESES lasting longer than 36 months had a normal language outcome. These data were used to support their recommendation that ESES should be terminated within 36 months to reduce the likelihood of long-term cognitive deficit. It should be pointed out that this important study has still not provided the answer to a key question in the management of children with ESES, namely what is the minimum duration of ESES that can result in permanent cognitive deficit? If clinicians knew the answer to this question it would give them a good indication of how long they might be prepared to wait for medical treatment to become effective before considering surgery. This is of major clinical importance because ESES seems to be quite resistant to medical treatment in many cases. Benzodiazepines, ACTH, steroids and valproate have all been tried. Some responses have been achieved. There is a lack of data on the effect of the new antiepileptic drugs on this condition, although lamotrigine can be highly successful in suppressing spike-wave discharges in other situations. If medical treatment is ineffective and the child has clearly lost skills in association with the ESES then surgery may be justified.

If the source of the ESES is a structural abnormality such as a porencephalic cyst, removal of the abnormality may resolve the ESES with consequent improvement in function. A novel surgical technique developed by Morrell (Morrell et al., 1989; Morrell et al., 1995) is multiple sub-pial transection. The underlying principle is that the surgeon transects the brain around the epileptic focus, preventing the spread of the epileptic discharges. This technique can be used in so-called 'eloquent' areas of brain, that is areas which, if resected, would result in unacceptable deficit.

Irwin *et al.* (2001) have recently reviewed the benefits of multiple sub-pial transection in five children, aged 5-10 years, with the Landau-Kleffner Syndrome. Both speech function and behaviour improved. The early work of Morrell revealed remarkable improvements in speech. Morrell *et al.* (1995) reported fourteen children with the Landau-Kleffner Syndrome who were treated with multiple sub-pial transection. Seven of these patients (50%) recovered age-appropriate speech and were educated in ordinary classes at school. These good results have not been replicated by some other groups, notably Mulligan *et al.* (2001) but this may reflect differences in pre-surgical selection criteria.

The interesting question relating to ESES is whether the epileptiform discharges themselves are responsible for the cognitive deterioration or whether the discharges are a manifestation of some other underlying degenerative process. Many workers now believe that the epileptiform discharges themselves, if allowed to continue for very long periods, cause permanent cognitive impairment. This appears to be supported by the evidence produced by workers such as Robinson *et al.* (2001) (see earlier section).

It might seem reasonable to advocate early aggressive treatment if a child shows clear cognitive deterioration and ESES is recorded in the EEG. However, some of these children may recover spontaneously, implying that the decision may not always be easy. In practice, it may be justifiable to allow the ESES to continue for weeks or months while every attempt is made to control it with medication. The ESES should certainly not be allowed to continue for as long as 36 months, as indicated by the analysis of Robinson *et al.* (2001).

If the condition has failed to respond to medical treatment and the child has clearly undergone cognitive deterioration then appropriate surgery, including, where necessary, multiple sub-pial transection, should be considered. Although, on one hand, it seems entirely appropriate to advocate early energetic intervention to prevent permanent cognitive impairment, on the other hand, some cases seem to resolve spontaneously and, in those cases, surgical treatment would not be justified. If there were reliable means of distinguishing between those who were likely to have a good prognosis without surgical treatment and those who were not, then the decision-making process would be much more straightforward.

(iv) Post-ictal effects of other epileptiform discharges.

Aldenkamp *et al.* (1996) have suggested that epileptiform discharges may have a post-ictal effect on cognitive function without causing transitory cognitive impairment. The current author (Besag, 2002) has recently discussed the findings.

Aldenkamp and colleagues compared four groups, aged 9-21 years: three with epilepsy and a control group. The first group had age-matched 'non-neurological' normal controls; the second group were patients with established epilepsy who had no epileptiform discharges or seizures during testing; the third group had epileptiform discharges but no detectable seizures over the period of testing and the fourth group had both epileptiform discharges and one or several seizures during the test sessions. It should be emphasised, however, that no obvious seizures occurred: the seizures were brief and subtle. They were only detected after extensive analysis of the video recordings. Patients and parents were unaware of these seizures. There were some possible confounding factors in this study, such as differences in the types of seizures and medication between the groups.

The results showed significant differences in the performance on intelligence subtests and tests of complex information processing between the control group and the fourth group, that is the group with both epileptiform discharges and subtle seizures. The authors discussed in some detail the possible reasons for these differences and concluded that they were probably the effects of both ictal and post-ictal changes.

It would have been of great interest if these authors could have shown an improvement in this particular group of subjects at other times when they were in another state with regard to the presence of subtle seizures or epileptiform discharges. Ideally this same group of people would have been tested in four states: with both discharges and subtle seizures, with subtle seizures and no discharges, with discharges but no subtle seizures and with neither discharges nor subtle seizures. Although this would have given a very informative set of test results, it is highly unlikely that these different states could all have been achieved in the same group of real patients.

CONCLUSION

It is very important to distinguish between permanent cognitive impairment and state-dependent, potentially reversible and treatable cognitive impairment; the EEG may be very helpful in making this distinction.

State-dependent cognitive impairment may be ictal or post-ictal, ongoing or transitory; the post-ictal form may be associated with daytime or night-time EEG abnormalities, including generalised or focal daytime seizures and electrical status epilepticus of slow wave sleep.

Any person who loses skills for no apparent reason, even if there is no history of seizures, deserves energetic investigation, including daytime and, if necessary, night-time EEG monitoring.

REFERENCES

Aarts, J.H., Binnie, C.D., Smit, A.M. and Wilkins, A.J. (1984). Selective cognitive impairment during focal and generalized epileptiform EEG activity. *Brain* **107**, 293-308.

Aldenkamp, A.P., Overweg, J., Gutter, T., Beun, A.M., Diepman, L. and Mulder, O.G. (1996). Effect of epilepsy, seizures and epileptiform EEG discharges on cognitive function. *Acta Neurol Scand* **93**, 253-259.

Beaumanoir, A. (1992). The Landau-Kleffner Syndrome. In: Roger, J., Bureau, M., Dravet, C., Dreifuss, F.E., Perret, A. and Wolf, P. (Eds), *Epileptic Syndromes in Infancy, Childhood and Adolescence.* John Libbey & Co Ltd, London, pp. 231-244.

Besag, F.M.C. (1994). Epilepsy education and the role of mental handicap. In: Ross, E.M. and Woody, R.C. (Eds), *Epilepsy.* Baillière Tindall, London, pp. 561-583.

Besag, F.M.C. (2001). Treatment of state-dependent learning disability. *Epilepsia* **42**, 52-54.

Besag, F.M.C. (2002). Childhood epilepsy in relation to mental handicap and behavioural disorders. *J Child Psychol Psychiatry* 43, 103-131.

Besag, F.M.C., Mills, M., Wardale, F., Andrew, C.M. and Craggs, M.D. (1989). The validation of a new ambulatory spike and wave monitor. *Electroencephalogr Clin Neurophysiol* 73, 157-161.

Binnie, C.D., Channon, S. and Marston, D. (1990). Learning disabilities in epilepsy: neurophysiological aspects. *Epilepsia* **31**, S2-S8.

Binnie, C.D., de Silva, M. and Hurst, A. (1992). Rolandic spikes and cognitive function. *Epilepsy Res* **6** (Suppl), 71-73.

Binnie, C.D. and Marston, D. (1992). Cognitive correlates of interictal discharges. *Epilepsia* **33**, S11-S17.

Cascino, G.D. (1993). Nonconvulsive status epilepticus in adults and children. *Epilepsia* **34** (Suppl 1), S21-S28.

Chugani, H.T. (1995). Infantile spasms. *Curr Opin Neurol* **8**, 139-144.

Chugani, H.T., Shewmon, D.A., Shields, W.D., Sankar, R., Comair, Y., Vinters H.V. and Peacock, W.J. (1993). Surgery for intractable infantile spasms: neuroimaging perspectives. *Epilepsia* **34**, 764-771.

de Menezes, M.A. and Rho, J.M. (2002). Clinical and electrographic features of epileptic spasms persisting beyond the second year of life. *Epilepsia* **43**, 623-630.

Dravet, C., Bueau, M., Guerrini, R., Giraud, N. and Roger J. (1992). Severe myoclonic epilepsy in infants. In: Roger, J., Bureau, M., Dravet, C., Dreifuss, F.E. Perret, A. and Wolf, P. (Eds.), *Epileptic Syndromes in Infancy, Childhood and Adolescence.* John Libbey & Co Ltd, London, pp. 75-88.

Gastaut, H., Roger, J., Soulayrol, R., Tassinari, C., Regis, H., Dravet, C., Bernard, C., Pinsard, N. and Saint-Jean, M. (1966). Childhood epileptic encephalopathy with diffuse slow spike-waves (otherwise known as 'petit mal variant') or Lennox syndrome. *Epilepsia* **7**, 139-179.

Goodman, R. (1986). Hemispherectomy and its alternatives in the treatment of intractable epilepsy in patients with infantile hemiplegia. *Dev Med Child Neurol* **28**, 251-258.

Irwin, K., Birch, V., Lees, J., Polkey, C., Alarcon, G., Binnie. C. *et al.* (2001). Multiple subpial transection in Landau-Kleffner syndrome. *Dev Med Child Neurol* **43**, 248-252.

Jambaqué, I., Chiron, C., Dumas, C., Mumford, J. and Dulac, O. (2000) Mental and behavioural outcome of infantile epilepsy treated by vigabatrin in tuberous sclerosis patients. *Epilepsy Res* **38**, 151-160.

Knight, E.S. and Oxbury, S.M. (2000). Cognitive and memory changes after hemispherectomy. In: Oxbury, J.M., Polkey, C.E. and Duchowny, M. (Eds), *Intractable Focal Epilepsy*. W B Saunders, Philadelphia, pp. 819-825.

Landau, W.M. and Kleffner, F.R. (1957). Syndrome of acquired aphasia with convulsive disorder in children. *Neurol (Minneap.)* **7**, 523-530.

Lindsay, J., Ounsted, C. and Richards, P. (1987). Hemispherectomy for childhood epilepsy: a 36-year study. *Dev Med Child Neurol* **29**, 592-600.

Marston, D., Besag, F., Binnie, C.D. and Fowler, M. (1993). Effects of transitory cognitive impairment on psychosocial functioning of children with epilepsy. A therapeutic trial: *Dev Med Child Neurol* **35**, 574-581.

Morrell, F., Whisler, W.W. and Bleck, T.P. (1989). Multiple subpial transection: a new approach to the surgical treatment of focal epilepsy. *J Neurosurg* **70**, 231-239.

Morrell, F., Whisler, W.W., Smith, M.C., Hoeppner, T.J. De, Toledo-Morrell, L., Pierre-

Louis, S.J., Kanner, A.M., Buelow, J.M., Ristanovic, R. and Bergen, D. (1995). Landau-Kleffner syndrome. Treatment with subpial intracortical transection. *Brain* **118**, 1529-1546.

Motte, J., Trevathan, E., Arvidsson, J.F., Barrera, M.N., Mullens, E.L. and Manasco, P. (1997). Lamotrigine for generalized seizures associated with the Lennox-Gastaut syndrome. Lamictal Lennox-Gastaut Study Group [published erratum appears in *N Engl J Med*, 1998, **339**, 851-852]. *N Engl J Med* **337**, 1807-1812.

Mulligan,L.P., Spencer, D.D. and Spencer, S.S. (2001). Multiple subpial transections: the Yale experience. *Epilepsia* **42**, 226-229.

Nieto-Barrera,M., Candau, R., Nieto-Jimenez, M., Correa, A. and Ruiz del Portal, L. (2000).Topiramate in the treatment of severe myoclonic epilepsy in infancy: *Seizure* **9**, 590-594.

Ohtahara, S., Ohtsuka, Y., Yamatogi, Y., Oka, E. and Inoue, H. (1992). Early infantile epileptic encephalopathy with suppression-bursts. In: Roger, J., Bureau, M., Dravet, C., Dreifuss, F.E., Perret, A. and Wolf, P. (Eds), *Epileptic Syndromes in Infancy, Childhood and Adolescence.* John Libbey & Co Ltd, London, p. 25-34.

Oxbury, S., Zaiwalla, Z., Adams, C., Middleton, J. and Oxbury, J. (1995). Hemispherectomy in childhood: serial neuropsychological follow-up and prolonged improvement. *Epilepsia* **36**, S24.

Patry, G., Lyagoubi, S. and Tassinari, C.A. (1971). Subclinical "electrical status epilepticus" induced by sleep in children. A clinical and electroencephalographic study of six cases: *Arch Neurol* **24**, 242-252.

Renier,W.O. (2000). West syndrome. In: Meinardi, H. (Ed), *Handbook of Clinical Neurology; The Epilepsies, Part II.* Elsevier, Amsterdam, pp. 199-210.

Robinson, R.O., Baird, G., Robinson, G. and Simonoff, E. (2001). Landau-Kleffner syndrome: course and correlates with outcome. *Dev Med Child Neurol* **43**, 243-247.

Ronen, G.M., Richards, J.E., Cunningham, C., Secord, M. and Rosenbloom, D. (2000). Can sodium valproate improve learning in children with epileptiform bursts but without clinical seizures? *Dev Med Child Neurol* **42**, 751-755.

Saint-Martin, A.D., Seegmuller, C., Carcangiu, R., Kleitz, C., Hirsch, E., Marescaux, C. and Metz-Lutz, M.N. (2001). [Cognitive consequences of Rolandic Epilepsy]. [French]: *Epileptic Disord 3 Spec No 2*, S159-S165.

Stores, G. and Hart, J.A. (1975). Proceedings: Reading skills of children with generalized and focal epilepsy attending ordinary school. *Electroencephalogr Clin Neurophysiol* **39**, 429-430.

Stores, G., Zaiwalla, Z., Styles, E. and Hoshika, A. (1995). Non-convulsive status epilepticus. *Arch Dis Child* **73**, 106-111.

Tassinari, C.A., Dalla, B.B. and Michelucci, R. (2000). Encephalopathy with electrical status epilepticus in slow sleep. In: Meinardi, H. (Ed), *Handbook of Neurology; The Epilepsies, Part II.* Elsevier, Amsterdam, pp. 267-280.

West, W.J. (1841). On a peculiar form of infantile convulsions. *Lancet* **i**, 724-725.

Westerveld, M., Sass, K.J., Chelune, G.J., Hermann, B.P., Barr, W.B., Loring, D.W., Strauss, E.,Trenerry, M.R., Perrine, K. and Spencer, D.D. (2000). Temporal lobectomy in children: cognitive outcome. *J Neurosurg* **92**, 24-30.

8

Ictally-Related Behavioural Syndromes that are Inter-Ictal in Nature: a Re-Evaluation of Epilepsy and Seizures

MICHAEL R. TRIMBLE

Institute of Neurology, UCL, National Hospital for Neurology and Neurosurgery, Queen Square, London and National Society for Epilepsy, Chalfont St Peter, Bucks

INTRODUCTION

Traditional classifications of the psychiatric disorders in epilepsy divide them into ictal and inter-ictal disorders. This goes back to the writings of the neuropsychiatrists of the 19th century, who made observations on patients with epilepsy, usually over the years, as they followed their progress often in an institutional setting. The division, between those syndromes driven by the ictus, and those that occur essentially independent of the ictus seems coherent, and has a certain degree of logic behind it. Further, it has allowed those who find associating epilepsy with psychiatry a difficult enterprise to identify a pragmatic division between what is neurological, i.e. seizure-related changes in behaviour, and what is psychiatric, namely those inter-ictal syndromes, of depression, anxiety, and personality disorder and psychoses. The former seem comprehensible in terms of the neurophysiological disturbances of the seizure. The latter became and remain areas of some controversy. While it may be the case that people with epilepsy develop, for example, psychoses, it is argued that this need not have anything to do with the neurophysiological disturbances of the epilepsy, but may relate to other factors, such as social pressures, chronic brain lesions, or the prescription of anti-epileptic drugs.

In recent years, there has been more agreement about the inter-ictal syndromes, and their biological associations with epilepsy. The Psychobiological

Commission of the International League Against Epilepsy (ILAE) has produced a consensus statement on classification (Krishnamoorthy and Trimble, 2002), which acknowledges that psychiatric disorders are frequent in patients with epilepsy, and they can be divided broadly into those that are simply co-morbid, and those that are likely to be biologically related to the epilepsy. The former are categorised essentially by one of the recognised diagnostic manuals, such as the DSM IV or the ICD 10. Thus, patients can have epilepsy, and panic disorder, and the two are viewed as independent (although acknowledging that patients with seizures get perhaps phobias and panic, linked through the psychological process of understandable fear of having, for example, seizures in public, or injuring themselves).

The other group of disorders are hypothesised to be more intimately woven with the biological process of the epilepsy, being viewed in part therefore as an, often albeit subtle, biological psycho-syndrome. These would include the inter-ictal dysphoric disorder (IDD) described by Blumer (2000), the inter-ictal personality disorder discussed by Geschwind and colleagues (Waxman and Geschwind, 1975) and the schizophrenia-like psychoses presented by Slater and Beard (1963).

This understanding of the behavioural presentations of epilepsy allows for a most important, but often overlooked feature of epileptology to be taken into account. Thus, the ILAE has developed a classification of epileptic syndromes, and another of epileptic seizures. This acknowledges that seizures and epilepsy are not the same, and require different conceptual approaches. It is in this context that the consideration of the ictal and inter-ictal can be reviewed. Thus the ictus (seizure) is but one manifestation of the epileptic process, and only a part of an epileptic syndrome. Further, it leaves open for debate as to what exactly the seizure is, and how it is to be defined. Clearly the seizure for a physician is an observable collation of clinical signs and symptoms, with some EEG changes, but for a neurophysiologist with electrodes placed in a hippocampal slice, it is an entirely different phenomenon.

Thus, the ictus, and what is ictal, peri-ictal, post-ictal and inter-ictal need careful consideration, and it is appropriate to revisit the simple earlier classifications that refer to inter-ictal and ictal as the primary caesura. Described here are two syndromes which are ictally related yet inter-ictal in presentation. They are not only clinically relevant, but also raise important conceptual issues about exactly what is epilepsy?

These two syndromes are clinically relevant to those looking after patients with learning disability, since they are often overlooked, but are predominantly behavioural in presentation. The first is the phenomenon referred to as forced normalisation, in which the seizural manifestation of the epilepsy is actually suppressed. The second are the post-ictal psychoses and related states, which occur after the clinical seizure has finished, and yet are related neurobiologically to the events of the seizure.

FORCED NORMALISATION

It was Landolt (1958) who noted that certain patients became psychotic when prescribed anti-epileptic drugs (AEDs) which suppressed their seizures. During the period of psychosis the EEG paradoxically normalised, losing its epileptic features. With the return of seizures, the EEG became abnormal again and the psychosis would resolve. Landolt used the term 'forced normalisation' to describe this phenomenon. 'Paradoxical normalisation' is another term (Wolf, 1991), which refers to the fact that the EEG during this state appears paradoxical. Thus, as a generalization, if a person has epilepsy and their behaviour deteriorates, the EEG also gets worse. For example if the patient develops a status epilepticus, or in the immediate post ictal phase of confusion, the EEG pattern is more abnormal than when the mental state is better. Further, if a patient develops more chronic behaviour changes, linked in with an organic brain syndrome (encephalopathy) the same is observed. However, in this singular setting of forced normalisation, the electroencephalogram improves dramatically as the behaviour worsens. It is paradoxical.

These are EEG terms; and the concept forced normalisation is essentially an EEG phenomenon. The accompanying clinical picture is better referred to as alternative psychosis, a name given by Tellenbach. It is now acknowledged that during these states the EEG does not have to normalise fully, or seizures cease completely.

These phenomena have become more frequent in recent times following the introduction of powerful anti-epileptic drugs (AEDs) which are given to patients with intractable seizures, and can render them seizure free quite quickly. The clinical pictures vary from paranoid psychoses resembling schizophrenia-like states, to episodes of irritability and conduct disturbance in children, to presentations with non-epileptic seizures. The majority of cases, however, are productive paranoid states, and require psychiatric intervention. Affective symptoms are frequently intermingled with the psychotic symptoms.

In patients with learning disability the disentanglement of the clinical picture can be very difficult, patients sometimes presenting with states of dysphoria, irritability and clinical withdrawal, and the actual psychosis not being readily apparent.

Treatment is either by removal of the AED with the resumption of seizures, or by prescription of neuroleptic or antidepressant medication, depending upon the clinical picture. Patients who have had an episode of alternative psychosis with one AED are susceptible to having it again with other drugs. In these cases it is advisable to start any new drug at low oral doses and increase the dose slowly, asking the patient or relatives to report any developing psychopathology.

PERI-ICTAL PSYCHOSES

This collection of behavioural changes related to the ictus includes ictal-psychoses, which are described briefly, but from the point of view of this text also the post-ictal psychoses and related presentations (Trimble, 1991).

Ictal psychoses. These are psychotic symptoms which occur as a direct reflection of the ictus and become prolonged, as in cases of non-convulsive status epilepticus, where the EEG reveals the diagnosis. Usually EEG studies performed during generalised (absence) status show generalised bilateral synchronous spike and wave activity, between 1-4 Hz. With complex partial seizure status, the EEG may show focal or bilateral epileptiform patterns with a slowing of the background. In these states, a wide range of psychopathology may be seen, including a mixture of abnormal affective and perceptual experiences, accompanied by automatisms, and fluctuating impaired consciousness. Amnesia would usually follow the episode.

Two types of complex focal status epilepticus are distinguished, a continuous form and a discontinuous or cyclical form. The latter consists of frequently recurring complex partial seizures. In between the seizures patients may or may not experience simple focal seizure symptoms, and consciousness may recover to near normal states.

A simple focal status, or *aura continua,* may lead to complex hallucinations, thought disorder and affective symptoms. In such cases, the continuous epileptic activity is often restricted, and may not even be detected with surface EEG recordings.

In an ictally-driven psychosis, the clinical picture may reveal fluctuating levels of consciousness, and a range of paranoid and schizophrenia-like symptoms.

POST-ICTAL PSYCHOSIS

These states have to be distinguished from the deliria which occur immediately post-ictally. In the latter, patients may often appear confused for up to 30 minutes, or sometimes longer following a seizure. They also sometimes report hallucinations but rarely delusions.

This is an organic brain syndrome which usually resolves spontaneously, but during which time the patient may become combative and may need subtle restraint.

The most common and best investigated peri-ictal psychosis, is that occurring post-ictally with as many as 18% of patients with intractable seizures being reported as experiencing one or more events in a lifetime of epilepsy.

The operational criteria for post-ictal psychosis are as follows:

1. onset of confusional psychosis within a week of the return of apparently normal mental function;

2. duration of between one day and three months;

3. a mental state characterised by a) clouding of consciousness, disorientation or delirium; b) delusions, hallucinations in clear consciousness; c) a mixture of a and b;

4. no evidence of factors which may have contributed to the abnormal mental state: a) anticonvulsant toxicity; b) a previous history of inter-ictal psychosis; c) EEG evidence of status epilepticus; d) recent head injury, or alcohol or drug intoxication.

The most quoted series is that of Logsdail and Toone (1988) who described 14 patients, the majority with complex partial seizures and secondary generalisation, in whom the psychosis developed after an exacerbation of the seizure activity, usually following a cluster of seizures.

Most had a lucid interval of up to 1-2 days, but sometimes longer, between the restoration of an apparently normal mental state following the seizure, and the beginning of the psychosis. The EEG during the post-ictal psychosis is variable, sometimes appearing relatively normal, in others showing an increase in abnormalities.

The range for the duration of the psychosis was up to 90 days, and many patients required psychotropic medication.

In their series, Logsdail and Toone followed patients for up to eight years and observed that the psychosis tended to recur. About 20% of patients go on to develop a chronic psychosis over time.

Of most interest is the lucid interval which is observed between the cessation of the seizures and the onset of the psychosis. Relatives describe this as the 'calm before the storm'. The psychosis, when it emerges, can be sudden and the behaviour can be extravagant; typically, hallucinations and delusions are noted, prominent are persecutory and religious phenomena. Most patients have at least partial recall for their psychotic experiences, and because the mental state is often not one of confusion, suicidal ideas, which occur in about one-fifth of patients, may be acted upon. Well directed violent attacks are seen in about 25% of episodes (Kanemoto *et al.*, 1996).

Post-ictal anxiety, like post-ictal depression, is not uncommon. Often it is biologically driven, as a feature of the temporal lobe syndrome, but it is also intertwined with fear of having further seizures, and the loss of confidence that goes with seizures in patients with intractable epilepsy. A self reinforcing situation can occur in which a patient, on account of seizures, is fearful of leaving the house in case they have a seizure, they become anxious and hyperventilate this can increase the chances of having further seizures.

Post-ictal depression. Post-ictal depression is not uncommon although its prevalence has never been estimated. It can last from hours to days and has features typical of a depressive syndrome. The density of the depression can be severe with some patients expressing suicidal thoughts. Suicide itself is not common unless associated with psychotic thinking.

There are a group of patients in whom post-ictal depression continues into a prolonged depressive illness and this becomes essentially an inter- ictal depression that requires antidepressant treatment (Robertson *et al.*, 1994).

In many settings, post-ictal depression accompanies the existential despair of patients who have intractable seizures, although biological components are clearly contributory, as are drug-related effects.

Treatment of ictally-related psychiatric disorders

A number of the psychopathologies discussed above are self limiting, and often no direct psychiatric intervention is required. The most problematic states are the post-ictal psychoses which can go on for several days. Since these patients can become suicidal and express paranoid delusions of consid- erable intensity, it is often important to prescribe psychotropic medication. Generally, it is better to avoid neuroleptics if possible, since they can lower the seizure threshold leading to further seizures and exacerbation of the psychosis. In the first instance, benzodiazepines are recommended. Clobazam can be used either to abort a cluster of seizures, by administering it immedi- ately after the initial seizure of a cluster, or after a cluster, with the first warning of any psychopathology. Relatives get to know the warning signs, which include irritability, sensitivity, mood lability and sleeplessness. If neuroleptic medications are to be used, those that lower the seizure threshold minimally are to be preferred. These include haloperidol, sulpiride and risperidone.

Obviously, crucial to the prevention of post-ictal psychosis is better control of the seizures. Post-ictal psychoses occurring in the setting of unilateral temporal lobe pathology are not a contra-indication for epilepsy surgery provided the patient has a very good chance of becoming seizure-free.

FURTHER OBSERVATIONS

The above disorders can represent a considerable diagnostic as well as clinical challenge, which is even more complicated in those with learning disability. Thus, while every one rejoices if a patient's seizure frequency declines significantly or they become seizure-free, but if this is at the expense of manageable behaviour, the balance may not be an acceptable one.

However, because of the benefit of having few or no seizures, and thence theoretically for the long-term outlook for the patient, there may be a reluc- tance to accept the link between the deteriorating behaviour and the thera- peutic success of the medication (or other treatment). Some practitioners simply do not accept the reality of the Landolt phenomenon, despite over half a century of clinical observations. Further, as noted, not all presentations are psychotic in a traditional psychiatric sense, and the behavioural picture can be quite polymorphic. Dysphoric irritability with increased hostility is a common presentation in the learning-disabled, behaviour sometimes attributed to an arousal or waking up of the patient with seizure-freedom, rather than as an alterative biological manifestation of a seizure.

It is often the case that such behaviours can be further controlled by judicious use of psychotropic medications, adding to polytherapy, but keeping the seizure frequency low (see Chapter 10). Careful discussions of the implications of different ways of handling patients with key personnel, care workers and the patients themselves are obviously very important.

The post-ictal states are frequently overlooked, sometimes because they are subtle in presentation (but severe enough to cause management problems), often because of the unrecognised lucid interval, but also because of their potential to be present almost continuously in a patient having several seizures a day. In other words, patients can remain ictal or post-ictal for much of the time. Only careful clinical observations, especially by carers and relevant key personnel, often combined with EEG studies will reveal the underlying clinical issues.

As noted in the introduction, part of the reluctance to recognise these seizure-related behavioural syndromes stems from a misunderstanding of the concepts of both epilepsy and seizures, and a failure to acknowledge the neurophysiological processes underlying them. These are related but substantially different, the seizure being but one manifestation of the enduring cerebral neuronal abnormalities underlying epilepsy. Given that these abnormalities are so frequently described in the limbic system, and that the latter is intimately related to the control of emotion and behaviour, alternative expressions of pathologies in that brain region are only to be expected.

CONCLUSIONS

In this chapter two syndromes which do not fit the traditional division of psychopathological disorders in epilepsy are described. Neither is clearly ictal or inter-ictal. The Landolt phenomenon is driven by suppression of the ictus, and can last as long as the suppression continues, while the post-ictal states can emerge several days after the seizure and last, on rare occasions, for weeks. And yet without the pathological processes underlying the seizure, neither would be possible. The links between such behavioural syndromes and epilepsy can hardly be denied, yet they challenge some of our concepts of what epilepsy is, or, for that matter, what a seizure is, and how they should be defined. From a clinical viewpoint, recognising and treating such behavioural syndromes can be a considerable challenge, often the more difficult in those with learning disability.

REFERENCES

Blumer, D. (2000). Dysphoric disorders and paroxysmal affects: recognition and treatment of epilepsy-related psychiatric disorders. *Harv Rev Psychiatry* **8**, 8-17.

Kanemoto, K., Kawasaki, J. and Kawai, I. (1996). Post ictal psychosis; a comparison with acute interictal and chronic psychoses, *Epilepsia* **37**,551-556.

Krishnamoorthy, E. S. and Trimble, M.R. (2002). Neuropsychiatric disorders in epilepsy – epidemiology and classification. In: Trimble, M.R. and Schmitz, B. (Eds), *The Neuropsychiatry of Epilepsy*. Cambridge University Press, Cambridge, pp 5 – 17.

Landolt, H.(1958). Serial electroencephalographic investigations during psychotic episodes in epileptic patients and during schizophrenic attacks. In: De Haas, Lorenz A. M. (Ed), *Lectures on Epilepsy*. Elsevier, Amsterdam pp 91-133.

Logsdail, S. and Toone, B.K. (l988). Post-ictal psychosis. A clinical and phenomenological description. *Br J Psychiatry* **152**, 246-252.

Robertson, M. M. Channon, S. and Baker, J. (1994). Depressive symptomatology in a general hospital sample of out patients with temporal lobe epilepsy: a controlled study. *Epilepsia* **35**,771-777.

Slater, E. and Beard, A.W.(1963). The schizophrenia-like psychoses of epilepsy. *Br J Psychiatry* **109**, 95-150.

Trimble, M.R. (1991). *The Psychoses of Epilepsy*. Raven Press, New York.

Waxman, S. G. and Geschwind, N. (1975). The interictal behaviour syndrome of temporal lobe epilepsy. *Arch Gen Psychiatry* **32**, 1580-1586.

Wolf.P. (1991). Acute behavioural symptomatology at disappearance of epileptiform EEG abnormality: paradoxical or forced normalisation. In: Smith, D. *et al*. (Eds), *Neurobehavioural Problems in Epilepsy: Advances in Neurology*. Raven Press, New York, pp 127-142.

Learning Disability and Epilepsy: an Integrative Approach
Edited by Michael R. Trimble
© 2003 Clarius Press Ltd

9

Anti-Epileptic Drug Treatments in Patients with Learning Disability

MIKE KERR

*University of Wales College of Medicine
Cardiff, UK*

INTRODUCTION

Clinicians working with people who have epilepsy and learning disability face special challenges when assessing the need for, and managing, drug interventions.

Conflicting concerns over medication side effects and seizure impact can be compounded by complex problems with communication and care provision. Furthermore, many individuals with a learning disability have difficult epilepsy syndromes that provide a significant therapeutic challenge.

Despite this, the situation for the clinician is clear in terms of therapeutic inputs. For the vast majority of individuals with a learning disability, epilepsy will be impacting on their lives and that of their carers, and thus they need treatment. For this population anti-epileptic drugs remain the cornerstone of treatments, notwithstanding the advances and improved accessibility of neurosurgical treatment.

This chapter, in addressing anti-epileptic drug treatments, will do so in the context of the skills and knowledge base necessary to provide management for this population. Such a knowledge base includes: (1) assessment of medication need, (2) principles of medication use, (3) treatment choice, and (4) assessment of treatment outcome.

ASSESSMENT OF MEDICATION NEED
– THE IMPACT OF EPILEPSY

The clinical decision to introduce antiepileptic medication is a balance between the potential medication side effects and an assessment of the impact of seizures on an individual. Uncontrolled seizures have a profound impact on the life of individuals and carers alike, irrespective of the presence of associated learning disability (Blunden, 1988; Brown *et al.*, 1993; Hoare, 1993; Vickrey, 1995; Espie *et al.*, 1998). Seizure disorders can have a broad range of negative impacts on: (1) the family, (2) behaviour and psychiatric disturbance, (3) physical morbidity and (4) mortality.

The Family

A range of factors associated with the impact of caring for an individual with a learning disability have been identified. These include: behaviour difficulties, the level of severity of learning disability, presence of multiple disabilities, and the level of social support (Eyman & Call, 1977; Bryne and Cunningham, 1985; Quine and Paul, 1985; Dunst *et al*, 1986; Carr, 1990; Orr *et al.*, 1991; Sloper *et al*, 1991; Heller *et al.*, 1997). The most consistently identified factor is the presence of a behavioural disturbance. Todd and Shearn (1996) provide some important pointers as to the problems experienced by carers in caring for someone with a learning disability. They found that families often regarded their offspring as a never-grown-up child and that carers organize their lives to meet care-giving needs.

Epilepsy also seems to be a factor associated with carer impact (Espie *et al.*, 1998). Unfortunately, however, we know surprisingly little about the precise impact of epilepsy on families of individuals who also have a learning disability. Levels of stress and dissatisfaction with their social situation were high, particularly in primary carers of a non-learning-disabled population with epilepsy (Thompson and Upton, 1992). Respite periods away from home were few and the perceived level of support was low. Poor emotional adjustment was associated with severity of tonic and atonic attacks and periods of status epilepticus, and low levels of support were associated with depression.

A study of children with epilepsy (Hoare, 1993) found the severity of the epilepsy and presence of learning and /or physical disabilities to be associated with carer impact. A qualitative survey of families caring for individuals with learning disability identified a significant carer 'burden' related to the epilepsy itself (Wilson, 1998). Carers experience strain, and family carers in particular may be prone to experience clinically significant levels of anxiety and depression (Espie *et al.*, 1998).

Behaviour and psychiatric problems

Considering the strong evidence for an increased prevalence of emotional disturbance in individuals with epilepsy who do not have learning disability (Hoare, 1984; Lund, 1985) it has proved much harder to find a similar link with people who have epilepsy and learning disability. Epidemiological evidence is not clear about such a population link in adults or children, as reviewed by Krishnamoorthy in Chapter 2. Some work (Espie *et al.*, 1989; Espie *et al.*, 1990) has shown that aggression and self-injury were associated with frequent seizures and polytherapy, but the absence of an epidemiological approach is almost certainly missing the potential for epilepsy to impact on individuals' patterns of behaviour. One question commonly arising in practice is that of whether an improvement in an individual's seizures can actually lead to deterioration in behaviour. It is rare to confirm such an association when detailed recordings are obtained, however this 'paradoxical normalisation' can occur and the underlying mechanisms may be similar to those seen in the clinical phenomenon of forced normalisation (Trimble and Schmitz, 1998).

Physical morbidity

Baxter (1999) found that people who had a learning disability and epilepsy had more admissions to accident and emergency than those who did not have epilepsy. It was also found that people with a learning disability and co-existing epilepsy have a much higher rate of fractures than those in the non-epilepsy learning disability population.

Mortality

Patients with epilepsy are known to have increased risk of mortality over the population in general (Cockerell *et al.*, 1994). Figures vary greatly, but range from a standardised mortality ratio (SMR) of 3 to over 7 in those aged under 20 (Shackleton *et al*, 1999; Nilsson *et al.*, 1997). This excess risk is partly explained by underlying causes of epilepsy such as cerebrovascular disease, injuries and poisoning. This probably explains the relatively higher SMRs in the year immediately after diagnosis of epilepsy (Cockerell *et al*, 1994).

People with a learning disability have a lower life expectancy than the general population (Forssman and Åkesson, 1970) with an estimated SMR of 1.6 (Forsgren *et al.*, 1996) and with measures likely to be indicative of the severity of learning disability, such as impaired mobility and incontinence, predicting early death (Hollins *et al.*, 1998).

This higher risk of mortality is increased for those patients with co-existing epilepsy (Forssman and Åkesson, 1970; Brorson and Wranne, 1987; Wieseler *et al.*, 1995; Forsgren *et al.*, 1996) whose SMR may be as high as 5.

In summary, the presence of epilepsy in a person with learning disability may well be impacting negatively on the lives of the individual and family alike. Active epilepsy with recurrent seizures will be a risk factor for mortality. Figure 1 highlights the assessment of epilepsy impact. In clinical settings it is usual to concur that the presence of continued seizures infers a continued risk from the impact of seizures. Such an assessment is likely to lead to the discussion of further therapeutic measures if these have not already been attempted.

Figure 1.   Assessing the impact of epilepsy.

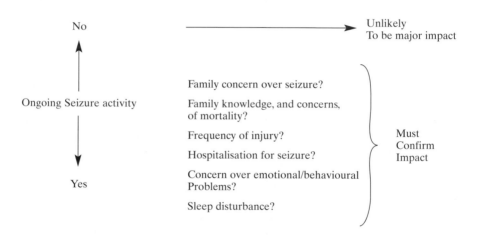

PRINCIPLES OF MEDICATION USE

Recent guidelines on the management of epilepsy in adults with a learning disability (IASSID Guidelines Group, 2001) highlight the following good practice principles in the use of anti-epileptic drugs:

I.   Ensure that the patient has received appropriate first-line treatment for their seizure type and syndrome.

II. In patients still continuing to have seizures, despite appropriate first-line anti-epileptic treatment:

   a. review diagnosis

   b. review treatment adherence

   c. ensure that the maximum tolerated dose has been used

III. If the first drug continues to be ineffective at the maximum tolerated dose, an alternative drug should be introduced slowly without tapering the first. If the patient has a good response to the second drug, then consider withdrawing the first drug gradually.

IV. If reasonable options for monotherapy have been explored and acceptable symptom control is still not achieved, long-term two-drug therapy should be tried.

V. If the first add-on drug is not effective, replace with a second add-on drug then slowly withdraw the ineffective drug. This process can be repeated for other possible add-on drugs.

VI. If symptoms are still not controlled on two drugs, some patients may benefit from an additional third drug.

TREATMENT CHOICE

Treatment choice should be driven by the available evidence base. For the treatment of epilepsy in people with a learning disability, this evidence base needs to be interrogated in a slightly different manner. The clinician will need to assess each drug, and therefore communicate this with the patient and carers on two levels. The first level involves data known from the non-learning disability population, and the second level involves data derived from learning disability related studies.

Furthermore, an analysis of certain characteristics of the drug which are particularly important to people with a learning disability should be assessed from the available non-learning disability studies. These characteristics include:

a. spectrum of action (partial, generalised or both);

b. drug interactions;

c. availability of varying preparations;

d. likely cognitive or behavioural side effects.

In order to address the issue of treatment choice, individual drug characteristics and clinical treatment scenarios will be discussed.

Individual drug characteristics

CARBAMAZEPINE

Indications: First line or adjunctive treatment in partial and generalised seizures (excluding absence and myoclonus).

Learning disability specific data: A randomised double blind placebo controlled comparison between the ordinary and the slow release preparation (SR) has been performed in learning disability (Kaski *et al.* 1991). This showed a potential efficacy advantage for SR when compared with usual carbamazepine.

Spectrum of action: As above, the potential to exacerbate myoclonus and absences is a significant problem in the complex, often cryptogenic generalised epilepsies in learning disability.

Drug interactions: significant inducer of hepatic enzymes with so many interactions possible.

Preparations: Tablets, chewtabs, liquid and suppository.

Likely cognitive or behavioural side effects: Known to be more cognitively impairing than lamotrigine; significant problem often on initiation.

CLOBAZAM

Indications: Adjunctive therapy for partial and generalised seizures. Intermittent short courses used for catamenial epilepsy and seizure deterioration.

Learning disability specific data: No trial data.

Spectrum of action: As above.

Drug interactions: Minor interactions may occur.

Preparations: Tablets, capsules.

Likely cognitive or behavioural side effects: Benzodiazepine side effects, drowsiness. Tolerable in short courses but regular therapy leads to tolerance of effect. Excessive salivation is major problem in learning disability.

CLONAZEPAM

Indications: Adjunctive therapy for partial and generalised seizures.

Learning disability specific data: No trial data.

Spectrum of action: As above.

Drug interactions: Minor interactions may occur.

Preparations: Tablets, liquid.

Likely cognitive or behavioural side effects: Benzodiazepine side effects, drowsiness. Tolerable in short courses but regular therapy leads to tolerance of effect. As with clobazam, excessive salivation is a major problem in learning disability.

ETHOSUXIMIDE

Indications: First line or adjunctive therapy in generalised absence seizures.

Learning disability specific data: No trial data.

Spectrum of action: As above.

Drug interactions: Levels reduced by enzyme inducing AEDs and increased by valproate.

Preparations: Capsules, syrup.

Likely cognitive or behavioural side effects: Plethora of behavioural and cognitive side effects mean caution needed when using in learning disability.

GABAPENTIN

Indications: Adjunctive treatment in partial and generalised seizures.

Learning disability specific data: An add-on comparative open study compared with lamotrigine in partial seizures (Crawford *et al.*, 2001) showed no difference between the two drugs (though underpowered).

Spectrum of action: Narrow spectrum.

Drug interactions: None.

Preparations: Capsules.

Likely cognitive or behavioural side effects: Well-tolerated, but released aggression has been reported.

LAMOTRIGINE

Indications: First line or adjunctive treatment in partial and generalised seizures and the Lennox Gastaut syndrome.

Learning disability specific data: A randomised double blind placebo controlled comparison in Lennox Gastaut syndrome showed efficacy with minimal impact of side effects (Motte *et al.*, 1997). An add-on comparative open study compared with gabapentin in partial seizures (Crawford *et al.*, 2001) showed no difference between the two drugs (though underpowered).

Spectrum of action: Broad spectrum; positive in learning disability, though caution is needed as it has been shown to exacerbate severe myoclonic epilepsy in some cases.

Drug interactions: Concentrations decreased by enzyme-inducing antiepileptic drugs. Levels increased when co-prescribed with sodium valproate.

Preparations: Tablets and chewtabs.

Likely cognitive or behavioural side effects: Has a very positive cognitive side effect profile and can, if anything, be slightly stimulating.

LEVETIRACETAM

Indications: Adjunctive therapy in partial seizures with or without secondary generalisation. Possible efficacy in generalised seizures though no current licence.

Learning disability specific data: No trial data available.

Spectrum of action: Broad spectrum; positive in learning disability, though caution is needed as off-licence use in generalised seizures is not currently supported by clinical trials.

Drug interactions: None.

Preparations: Tablets.

Likely cognitive or behavioural side effects: Has a positive cognitive side effect profile in non-learning disability subjects.

OXCARBAZEPINE

Indications: Adjunctive or monotherapy treatment in partial seizures with or without secondary generalisation.

Learning disability specific data: As yet no trial data available.

Spectrum of action: Narrow spectrum; likely to be similar problems to carbamazepine.

Drug interactions: Similar but fewer than with carbamazepine.

Preparations: Tablets.

Likely cognitive or behavioural side effects: Similar though to a lesser extent than carbamazepine.

PHENOBARBITAL

Indications: Adjunctive or monotherapy use in partial or generalised seizures.

Learning disability specific data: No trial data available.

Spectrum of action: Broad.

Drug interactions: Enzyme induction leads to many potential drug interactions.

Preparations: Tablets, elixir, injection.

Likely cognitive or behavioural side effects: Very poor cognitive profile, not recommended except in exceptional circumstances due to significant risk of behavioural difficulties and somnolence.

PHENYTOIN

Indications: Adjunctive or monotherapy use in partial or generalised seizures (excluding myoclonus and absence).

Learning disability specific data: No trial data available.

Spectrum of action: Broad but no efficacy in myoclonus or absences.

Drug interactions: Enzyme induction leads to many potential drug interactions.

Preparations: Capsules, chewtabs, liquid suspension, and injection.

Likely cognitive or behavioural side effects: Poor cognitive profile, not recommended except in exceptional circumstances due to significant risk of cognitive side effects.

PRIMIDONE

Indications: Adjunctive or monotherapy use in partial or secondarily generalised seizures.

Learning disability specific data: No trial data available.

Spectrum of action: As above.

Drug interactions: Enzyme induction leads to many potential drug interactions.

Preparations: Tablets, liquid suspension.

Likely cognitive or behavioural side effects: Poor cognitive profile, not recommended except in exceptional circumstances due to significant risk of cognitive side effects.

TIAGABINE

Indications: Adjunctive therapy in partial or secondarily generalised seizures.

Learning disability specific data: No trial data available.

Spectrum of action: Restricted to partial epilepsy.

Drug interactions: Enzyme induction leads to reduction in tiagabine levels.

Preparations: Tablets.

Likely cognitive or behavioural side effects: Generally good profile but dose-related effects causing dizziness and anxiety could limit use of effective dosages.

TOPIRAMATE

Indications: Adjunctive therapy in partial, secondarily generalised, primary generalised seizures and in Lennox Gastaut syndrome.

Learning disability specific data: A randomised placebo controlled trial in Lennox Gastaut showed efficacy in atonic seizures (Sachdeo *et al.*, 1996).

Spectrum of action: Broad.

Drug interactions: Enzyme induction leads to reduction in topiramate levels.

Preparations: Tablets, sprinkle.

Likely cognitive or behavioural side effects: Has potential for significant cognitive side effects particularly in dose escalation. Slow dose titration needed. Usually this will avoid major difficulties. Weight loss can be a problem in those already underweight.

VALPROATE

Indications: First line and adjunctive therapy in partial and generalised seizures.

Learning disability specific data: No trial data available.

Spectrum of action: Broad.

Drug interactions: When used with lamotrigine causes an increase in lamotrigine levels.

Preparations: Tablets, slow release tablets, crushable tablets, liquid and sprinkle.

Likely cognitive or behavioural side effects: Generally well tolerated, weight gain can be a significant problem.

VIGABATRIN

Indications: Adjunctive therapy in partial and secondarily generalised seizures.

Learning disability specific data: Some prospective follow up studies (Matilainen *et al.*, 1988; Pitkanen *et al.*, 1993) show good efficacy and tolerability.

Spectrum of action: As above.

Drug interactions: May lower phenytoin levels.

Preparations: Tablets, powder sachets.

Likely cognitive or behavioural side effects: Potential for significant behavioural changes. Known to cause severe visual field restriction and therefore use now very limited.

CLINICAL TREATMENT SCENARIOS

People with a learning disability who have epilepsy will encounter the same clinical treatment scenarios as their non-learning-disabled counterparts. These will include:

1. Initial monotherapy

2. New add-on drugs in treatment failure

3. Treatment of prolonged and cluster seizures

Initial monotherapy

Monotherapy treatment decisions should be made in consultation with the individual and the carers. Table 1 highlights the possible monotherapy choices for both partial and generalised seizures.

Clinicians should be very careful to balance the assessment of a person with learning disability as having all the needs of the non-disabled patient with epilepsy, whilst recognising the potential both for specific sensitivity to side effects that are hard to communicate and for cognitive side effects.

Table 1.   Monotherapy choices for people with a learning disability.

Generalised seizures	Partial seizures
Lamotrigine, Sodium Valproate*	Carbamazepine, Lamotrigine**, Sodium Valproate*
*In women of childbearing potential the relative risks of all AEDs to the unborn child should be discussed	**A comparative trial of lamotrigine and carbamazepine identified a favourable side effect profile for lamotrigine.

Figure 2.   Treatment pathways following drug failure.

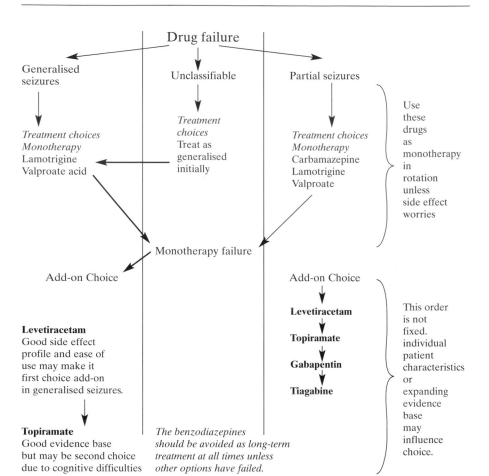

New add-on drugs in treatment failure

The likelihood of drug change is almost certainly increased for people with a learning disability, given their propensity to more severe seizure disorders. Therefore, clinicians treating epilepsy in the population must have at hand a good knowledge of all available anti-epileptic drugs. Figure 2 describes a treatment pathway following drug failure. Crucial in this process is an appropriate identification of drug failure – insufficient seizure control and/or unacceptable side effects. It is also important to see this process as dynamic and life-long with decisions being made over time and the decision to make a change varying over time.

Treatment of prolonged and cluster seizures

Individuals who have epilepsy and learning disability often have a need for treatments for prolonged or cluster seizures. Good evidence exists for the use of diazepam by oral or rectal use and some evidence is appearing for the use of buccal or intranasal midazolam. Such treatments need clear and precise guidelines for their administration. This is particularly true for this population, where individuals often have a varied and rapidly changing care setting, which increases the potential for drug error. Therefore a structured plan for the administration of such rescue medication is essential. Such a plan should include the following basic standards:

• Any individual who has epilepsy and learning disability should have an assessment of the management of prolonged seizures and/or cluster seizures;

• Where rescue medication is prescribed, a care plan should be completed which must include:

  • drug type and dose,

  • duration of seizure before administration,

  • timing before repeat administration,

  • maximum dosage in 24 hours,

  • advice on when to call for an ambulance.

ASSESSMENT OF TREATMENT OUTCOME

In the usual practice of epileptology, an assessment of treatment outcome is a clinical decision made with the patient. This decision is a composite of several factors including: (1) whether the seizure control is acceptable, (2) whether side effects are tolerable, and (3) potential lifestyle implications to the patient, such as if change is necessary due to an aim to have a family.

Secondary to this, a range of measures is used to analyse outcome in experimental, or quasi-experimental, situations. These include: (a) seizure frequency, (b) seizure severity, and (c) quality of life measures. Seizure severity measures have not been validated in people with learning disabilities (Kerr and Espie, 1997). Furthermore, quality of life measures designed for non-learning disability patients may not be relevant.

The clinician dealing with people with learning disability and epilepsy will need to have an understanding of those *measures used in research* whilst, understandably, having a more pragmatic approach to *clinic-based assessment.*

Measures used in research

The growing number of quality of life measures designed to evaluate the lifestyle of people with learning disabilities (Cummins, 1997) have not been validated as outcomes in epilepsy management.

However, there is an increasing amount of research that has acknowledged a combination of measures used in learning disability research, including general healthcare research and new measures designed specifically for people with a learning disability who have epilepsy.

Espie *et al.* (1997) have stressed three key components to outcome, the first being *defining the individual patient*. This may be approached by assessment of several variables, including: ability defined using such rating scales as the Adaptive Behaviour Scale (Nihira *et al.*, 1993); personal attributes where specific traits such as behaviour could be measured using such scales as the Aberrant Behaviour Checklist (Aman and Singh, 1983); aetiology; seizure syndrome.

The second area involves the use of *measures that are sensitive to change* to determine the efficacy of a treatment in a specific patient. Seizure diaries are helpful to clinicians in diagnosis and treatment (Espie and Paul, 1997). The Liverpool Seizure Severity Scale has been adapted for people with learning disabilities and has good reliability (Espie *et al.*, 1997). Other appropriate measures include: seizure frequency – which may be recorded on a seizure chart; behaviour – monitored by a scale such as the Aberrant Behaviour Checklist (Aman and Singh, 1983); social interaction; patient independence; and contact and participation – assessed by direct observation; general well-being – monitored on a global scale involving the targeting of certain baselines such as sleep or appetite, or a parent's or carer's view of how the patient is and whether a certain variable has changed over time.

The third area is the measurement of the effect of the patient's epilepsy on their carers. Here, in the absence of validated epilepsy related scales, generic quality of life measures such as the SF 36 and the Malaise Care-giver Index (Rutter *et al.*, 1970) or specific trait measures such as the Beck Depression Inventory (Beck and Steer, 1997) could be employed. Also specific intellectual disability and epilepsy scales have been developed such as the Epilepsy Outcome Scale (Espie *et al.*, 1998). A further scale, the Epilepsy and Learning Disability Quality of Life Scale (Jacoby *et al.*, 1996), has been applied in pharmacological research.

Characteristics of carers, as well as those of patients, may also influence outcome. Jarvie and colleagues have developed a questionnaire to assess knowledge of epilepsy (Jarvie *et al.*, 1993). They state that knowledge of epilepsy plays a vital role in a person's ability to cope successfully with this condition, and misconceptions about the condition can lead to unnecessary recreational restrictions. Therefore they suggest that the development of this

Figure 3. Assessing behavioural change during antiepileptic drug treatment.

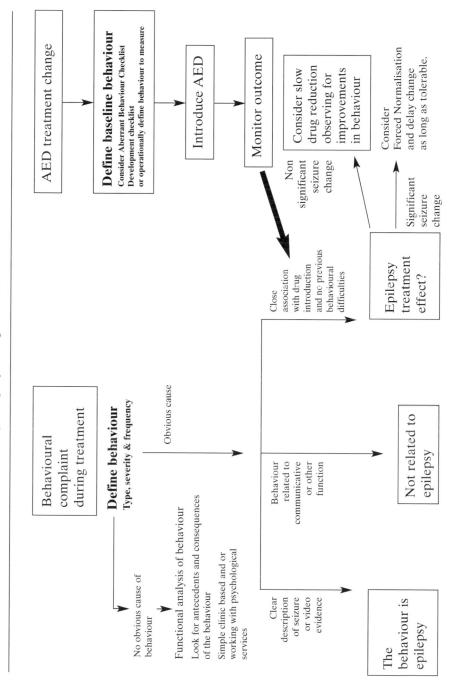

measure could prove invaluable in both clinical and non-clinical settings for the care and treatment of people with epilepsy.

Clinic-based assessment

Despite these increasingly elegant measures designed to analyse the outcome of our interventions, it is likely that in a clinical context the assessment of treatment outcome will involve a more pragmatic approach. This approach is likely to have several broad aims. The first will be to analyse accurately any seizure change. To do this, accurate seizure charts are necessary. These will need space to identify several seizure types. Acquiring high-quality seizure frequency data can be a long-term and difficult process. Frequently parents and carers will need guidance in differentiating varying seizure types and in accurate recording. Clinicians may have to work with other members of the team, such as specialist nurses or community learning disability nurses, to aid in this process.

Secondly, clinicians will have to assess any negative impact from the treatment change. This again can be a challenging task, especially in individuals who may have poor communication skills and a range of concurrent illnesses all with symptoms not unlike those of potential drug side effects. Of these, of most concern to clinicians and carers alike is the potential for behaviour change. A structured approach is necessary to identify those occasions where behavioural symptoms are likely to be treatment-related (see Figure 3).

Lastly, the decision on treatment outcome is dependent on an accurate assessment and discussion of all these factors with the patient and carers. This must be informed decision making, with patients and carers being as informed of the risks of continued seizures as they may be of drug side effects.

CONCLUSION

The use of anti-epileptic medication in people with learning disability remains the most significant option to reduce the very significant morbidity caused by epilepsy in this population. High clinical skill and competency is needed for successful use of medication. The arrival of a range of novel antiepileptic drugs has greatly increased patient options; the challenge is to expose patients to these new options in a skilled and professional manner.

REFERENCES

Aman, M. and Singh, N. (1983). Pharmacological intervention. In: Matson, J. and Mulick, J. (Eds), *Handbook of Mental Retardation*. Pergamon, New York, pp. 317-337.

Baxter, H.A, (1999). Personal communication.

Beck, A.T. and Steer, R.A. (1997). *The Beck Depression Inventory: Manual*. The Psychological Corporation, San Antonio, Texas.

Blunden, R. (1988). Pragmatic features of quality services. In: Janicki, M.P., Krauss, M.W. and Seltzer, M.M. (Eds), *Community Residences for Persons with Developmental Disabilities: Here to Stay*. Paul H. Brookes, Baltimore.

Brorson, L.O. and Wranne, L. (1987). Long-term prognosis in childhood epilepsy: survival and seizure prognosis. *Epilepsia* **28**, 324-330.

Brown, S.W., Betts, T.A., Chadwick, D. *et al.* (1993). An epilepsy needs document. *Seizure* **2**, 91-103.

Bryne, E. and Cunningham, C. (1985). The effects of mentally handicapped children on families. A conceptual review. *J Child Psychol Psychiatry* **26**, 847-864.

Carr, J. (1990). Supporting families of people with behavioural / psychiatric difficulties. *Int Rev Psychiatry* **2**, 33-42.

Cockerell, O.C., Johnson, A.L., Sander, J.W.A.S., Hart, Y.M. and Goodridge, D.M.G. (1994). Mortality from epilepsy: results from a prospective population-based study. *Lancet* **344**, 918-921.

Crawford P., Brown S. and Kerr M. (2001). A randomized open-label study of gabapentin and lamotrigine in adults with learning disability and resistant epilepsy. *Seizure* **10**, 107-115.

Cummins, R.A. (1997). Assessing Quality of Life. In: Brown R.I. (Ed.), *Quality of Life for People with Disabilities, 2nd Edition*. Stanley Thornes (Publishers) Ltd, London, pp.116-150.

Dunst, C., Trivette, C. and Cross, A. (1986). Mediating influences of social support: personal, family and child outcomes. *Am J Ment Def* **90**, 403-417.

Espie, C.A., Pashley, A.S., Bonham, K.G., Sourindhrin, I. and O'Donovan, M. (1989). The mentally handicapped person with epilepsy: a comparative study investigating psychosocial functioning. *J Ment Def Res* **33**, 123-135.

Espie, C.A., Gillies, J.B. and Montgomery, J.M. (1990). Antiepileptic polypharmacy, psychosocial behaviour and locus of control orientation among mentally handicapped adults living in the community. *J Ment Def Res* **34**, 351-360.

Espie, C.A., Kerr, M., Paul, A., O'Brien, G., Betts, T., Clark, J., Jacoby, A. and Baker, G. (1997). Learning disability and epilepsy. 2: A review of available outcome measures and position statement on development priorities. *Seizure* **6**, 337-350.

Espie, C.A. and Paul, A. (1997). Epilepsy and learning disability. In: Goldstein, L. and Cull, C. (Eds.) *The Clinical Psychologist's Handbook of Epilepsy*. Routledge, London, pp. 184-202.

Espie, C.A., Paul, A., Graham, M. *et al.* (1998). The Epilepsy Outcome Scale: the development of a measure for use with carer's of people with epilepsy plus intellectual disability. *J Intellect Disabil Res* **42**, 90-96.

Eyman, R.K. and Call, T. (1977). Maladaptive behaviour and community placement of mentally retarded persons. *Am J Ment Retard* **82**, 137-144.

Forsgren, L., Edvinsson, S., Nystrom, L. and Blomquist, H.K. (1996). Influence of epilepsy on mortality in mental retardation: an epidemiological study. *Epilepsia* **37**, 956-963.

Forssman, H. and Åkesson, H.O. (1970). Mortality of the mentally deficient: a study of 12,903 institutionalised subjects. *J Ment Def Res* **14**, 276-294.

Heller, T., Miller, A. and Factor, A. (1997). Adults with mental retardation as supports to their parents: Effects on parental caregiving appraisal. *Ment Retard* **35**, 338-346.

Hoare, P. (1984). The development of psychiatric disorder among school children with epilepsy. *Dev Med Child Neurol* **26**, 3-13.

Hoare, P. (1993). The quality of life of children with chronic epilepsy and their families. *Seizure* **2**, 269-275.

Hollins, S., Attard, M.T., von Fraunhofer, N., McGuigan, S. and Sedgewick, P. (1998). Mortality in people with learning disability: risk, causes and death certification findings in London. *Dev Med Child Neurol* **40**, 50-56.

IASSID Guidelines Group. (2001). Clinical guidelines for the management of epilepsy in adults with an Intellectual Disability. *Seizure* **10**(6), 401-409.

Jacoby, A., Baker. G., Bryant-Constock, L., Phillips, S. and Bamford, C. (1996). Lamotrigine add-on therapy is associated with improvement in mood in patients with severe epilepsy. *Epilepsia* **37** (Suppl. 5), 202.

Jarvie, S., Espie, C.A., and Brodie, M.J. (1993). The development of a questionnaire to assess knowledge of epilepsy: 1. General knowledge of epilepsy. *Seizure* **2**, 179-185.

Kaski, M., Heineken, E., Seventies, J., Tommie, J. and Attila, M. (1991). Treatment of epilepsy in mentally retarded patients with a slow-release carbamazepine preparation. *J Ment Def Res* **35**, 231-239.

Kerr, M.P. and Espie, C.A. (1997). Learning disabilities and epilepsy. 1: Towards common outcome measures. *Seizure* **6**, 331-336.

Lund, J. (1985). Epilepsy and psychiatric disorder in the mentally retarded adult. *Acta Psychiatr Scand* **72**, 557-562.

Matilainen, R., Pitkänen, A., Ruutiainen, T., Mervaala, E., Sarlund, H. and Riekkinen P. (1988). Effect of vigabatrin on epilepsy in mentally retarded patients: a seven-month follow-up study. *Neurology* **38**, 743-747.

Motte, J., Trevathan, E., Barrera, M.N., Mullens, E.L. and Manasco, P. (1997). Lamotrigine for generalized seizures associated with the Lennox-Gastaut syndrome. *N Engl J Med* **337**, 1807-1812.

Nihira, K., Leland, H. and Lambert, N. (1993). *Adaptive Behaviour Scales.* American Association on Mental Retardation. Austin, Texas.

Nilsson, L., Tomson, T., Farahmand, B.Y., Diwan, V. and Persson, P.G. (1997). Cause-specific mortality in epilepsy: a cohort study of more than 9,000 patients once hospitalised for epilepsy. *Epilepsia* **38**, 1062-1068.

Orr, R., Cameron, S. and Day, D. (1991). Coping with stress in families with children who have mental retardation: An evaluation of the double ABCX model. *Am J Ment Retard* **95**, 444-450.

Pitkänen, A., Ylinen, A., Matilainen, R., Luukkainen, R., Mervaala, E., Seppanen, R., Ruutiainen, T. and Riekkinen, P.J. (1993). Long-term anti-epileptic efficacy of vigabatrin in drug-refractory epilepsy in mentally retarded patients. A 5-year follow-up study. *Arch Neurol* **50**, 24-29.

Quine, L and Paul, L. (1985). Examining the causes of stress in families with severely handicapped children. *Br J Soc Work* **15**, 501-517.

Rutter, M., Tizard, J. and Whitmore, K. (1970). *Education, Health and Behaviour.* Longmans, London.

Sachdeo, R., Kugler, S., Wenger, E. and Mandelbaum, D. (1996). Topiramate in Lennox Gastaut syndrome. *Epilepsia* **37**, 118.

Shackleton, D.P., Westendorp, R.G.J., Kasteleijn-Nolst Trenite, D.G.A. and Vandenbroucke, J.P. (1999). Mortality in patients with epilepsy: 40 years of follow up in a Dutch cohort study. *J Neurol Neurosurg Psychiatry* **66**, 636-640.

Sloper, P., Knussen, C. and Turner, S. (1991). Factors related to stress and satisfaction in families of children with Down's syndrome. *J Child Psychol Psychiatry* **32**, 655-676.

Thompson, P.J. and Upton, D. (1992). The impact of chronic epilepsy on the family. *Seizure* **1**, 43-48.

Todd, S. and Shearn, J. (1996). Struggles with time: the careers of parents with adult sons and daughters with learning disabilities. *Disabil Society* **11**, 379-401.

Trimble, M.R. and Schmitz, B. (1998). *Forced Normalisation and the Alternative Psychoses of Epilepsy*. Wrightson Biomedical Publishing, Petersfield.

Vickrey, B.G. (1995). Advances in the measurement of health-related quality of life in epilepsy. *Qual Life Res* **4**, 83-85.

Wieseler, N.A., Hanson, R.H. and Nord, G. (1995). Investigation of mortality and morbidity associated with severe self-injurious behaviour. *Am J Ment Retard* **100**, 1-5.

Wilson, R. (1998). *Unpublished MSc Thesis*. University of Wales College of Medicine.

ACKNOWLEDGEMENT

I would like to thank my colleagues with whom several of the ideas in this chapter have been developed. In particular Ms Helen Baxter, Claire Smith and Dr Mark Scheepers.

Learning Disability and Epilepsy: an Integrative Approach
Edited by Michael R. Trimble
© 2003 Clarius Press Ltd

10

On the Use of Psychotropic Drugs in Patients with Learning Disability and Epilepsy

MICHAEL R. TRIMBLE

Institute of Neurology, Queen Square, London, UK

INTRODUCTION

It is now accepted that many patients with epilepsy have psychiatric problems, and recent epidemiological evidence from selected clinics suggest that over 50% of patients may have a recognisable psychiatric disorder (Krishnamoorthy and Trimble, 2002). It is also known that many patients with epilepsy receive psychotropic drugs, sometimes, but not always, on account of their psychiatric symptoms. Thus, it has to be acknowledged that there is a careful overlap between anticonvulsant drugs and psychotropic agents, such that many of the former are known to have mood regulating properties, while a number of the latter (for example: benzodiazepines) have anticonvulsant properties.

The situation in patients with learning disability is similar, with the exception that diagnostic issues are more complicated, and, in many instances, psychotropic agents are used to suppress unwanted behaviours, such as aggression, but in the absence of a clear diagnostic formulation. The most commonly used drugs in the learning disabled population are neuroleptics, which are prescribed for up to 60% of patients (Sachdev, 1992).

Generally, patients with learning disability, particular with more severe disablement, who also have epilepsy are at an additional risk for the development of behaviour problems. There is the risk that goes with learning disability, plus the additional complications of the feedback from seizures, often with poor seizure control, and the problems of medication. However, as with the studies of anticonvulsant medications in this population, there is very little in the way of double-blind controlled or even placebo controlled studies of the use of psychotropic drugs, the majority of data coming from

Phase 4 open studies. Most of this work has been carried out in people who do not have epilepsy, or in populations in which the percentage of patients with epilepsy is not well specified.

The majority of this text discusses antidepressant and antipsychotic drugs, with some further brief comments about other psychotropic drugs that are also used in the management of behaviour problems. A classification of psychotropic drugs currently in use is given in Table 1.

Table 1. Classification of psychotropic drugs

Antidepressants

Antipsychotics

Minor tranquillisers

Mood stabilisers

Psychostimulants

Others (beta blockers etc.)

ANTIDEPRESSANT DRUGS, SEIZURES AND EPILEPSY

Ever since the introduction of tricyclic antidepressant drugs into clinical practice, seizures have been recognised as a side effect. This has been reviewed on several occasions (Trimble, 1980; 1987). The position has changed in the last few years because of the introduction of a number of new antidepressant drugs, and following a brief review of the older literature, these will be discussed.

A review of some early studies

Animal data

A number of laboratory and clinical investigations were carried out to assess the effect of tricyclic antidepressants on seizures and the seizure threshold. The early laboratory investigations essentially revealed the proconvulsant effect of these agents, and it emerged from these studies that clomipramine, amitriptyline, and maprotiline were probably the most proconvulsant compounds (Trimble, 1987).

Luchins *et al.*, (1984) used spike activity in perfused guinea pig hippocampal slices as an indication of epileptogenicity and reported the effect of a variety of antidepressants. Imipramine, amitriptyline, nortriptyline, desipramine and maprotiline generally increased spike activity, while viloxazine, protriptyline and trimipramine appeared to decrease neuronal excitability. Some agents, for example, doxepin produced a significant increase in excitability, and then with higher dose significant decreases, suggesting a biphasic effect. In this model mianserin had no effect.

Using the photosensitive baboon, *Papio papio*, Trimble *et al.*, (1977) compared two tricyclic drugs, namely clomipramine and imipramine, and the quadricyclic drug maprotiline with the non-tricyclic nomifensine. The first three all lowered the seizure threshold, while nomifensine had little effect and in some animals was anticonvulsant.

One interesting drug examined in these early studies was viloxazine. In two animal models (Luchins *et al.*, 1984; Meldrum *et al.*, 1982) it was observed, if anything, to have a seizure-protective effect.

These early animal studies therefore suggested the potential for both anticonvulsant and proconvulsant effects of these drugs, and with some compounds there was evidence of a dose-related effect.

Clinical data

The clinical data at that time came mainly from reports of government agencies such as the Committee on Safety of Medicines, and from clinical trials. Several reviews emphasised the poor quality of the available information (Edwards, 1985). However, from the clinical studies the highest reporting of seizures was with maprotiline and clomipramine, and the lowest reporting with protriptyline.

The estimated risk of seizures with tricyclic drugs was around 0.06 to 0.1% (Burley, 1977; Jick *et al.*, 1983). The incidence of seizures with imipramine was 0.7%, and with clomipramine 3.0%.

Garvey and Tollefson (1987) drew attention to myoclonic seizures that could occur in relation to tricyclic antidepressant drug prescribing, and suggested that as many as 40% of patients reported some kind of myoclonic event after starting them. They calculated the frequency of the effect with the different drugs in descending order from maprotiline, trazodone, nortriptyline, desimpramine, amitriptyline to imipramine. Dothiepin was not associated with this effect.

Other information that emerged from the early clinical studies was the low reporting of seizures with viloxazine (Edwards and Glen-Bott, 1984), and, for proconvulsant drugs, a relationship of seizure-reporting to the therapeutic dose. Higher doses of the drug have a higher frequency of seizures, a clear relationship to overdose. There was a relationship of seizures to the number of different psychotropic drugs prescribed.

The time relationship between commencing the drug and the seizures varies considerably between studies. The attack may occur from 24 hours to several weeks after starting an antidepressant, although early seizures (less than a week) would seem to be associated with lower dosing schedules and possibly more patient-related factors that lower the seizure threshold than later onset seizures (Trimble, 1980).

It was generally concluded that patients were more likely to have seizures (if they did not have epilepsy) if they had a family history of seizures, or a past history of relevant medical conditions such as a head injury or a cerebrovascular accident.

Few of the above antidepressant drugs were tried in patients with epilepsy. Viloxazine was studied, but it was shown to lead easily to anticonvulsant drug toxicity, and was therefore not recommended in epilepsy (Pisani *et al.*, 1984).

Paradoxically, there were some clinical reports of tricyclic antidepressants being anticonvulsant. Ojemann and colleagues reported retrospective data, which suggested that doxepin improved seizure frequency in 15 of 19 patients who were prescribed the drug (Ojemann *et al.*, 1983). This included a diminution of both partial and generalised tonic-clonic seizures.

Conclusions from these earlier clinical studies were that, in general, antidepressant drugs were proconvulsant, although they were not all proconvulsant to the same degree, and some may not alter the seizure threshold or have a biphasic effect, sometimes revealing some anticonvulsant effects. Table 2 shows factors which were thought to be interlinked with lowering of the seizure threshold, emphasising that this is a problem of the use of these drugs which is not confined to epilepsy. There are many patients without epilepsy, who have a lowered seizure threshold, who are susceptible to psychotropic-induced seizures.

Table 2.   Factors that lower the seizure threshold

A family history of epilepsy
Head injury, especially with a prolonged post-traumatic amnesia, or intracranial injury
Neurological illness

Newer antidepressant drugs

There have been several developments of antidepressants since the tricyclic era. Some drugs have been mentioned briefly above, which were nontricyclic, such as mianserin, maprotiline and viloxazine. However, the major development in the last few years has been of agents that selectively inhibit the re-uptake of either noradrenaline, or serotonin, or both.

In brief, the selective serotonin re-uptake inhibitors (SSRIs) are represented by citalopram, fluoxetine, fluvoxamine, sertraline and paroxetine. Of these, citalopram is the most selective on serontonin re-uptake, inhibiting serotonin re-uptake 3,000 times more than noradrenaline uptake, and 22,000 times more than dopamine (Noble and Benfield, 1997). In general, the SSRIs are better tolerated and safer in overdose compared to tricyclic drugs.

Table 3.   Newer antidepressants

Noradrenergic uptake inhibitors – reboxetine
Serotonin-noradrenaline uptake inhibitors - venlafaxine
Serotonin antagonist/reuptake inhibitor – nefazodone
Noradrenaline-selective serotonin uptake inhibitors - mirtazapine

Table 4.   Receptor profile and epileptogenic potential of antidepressants

Drug	Action on receptor						Seizures/epilepsy
	H_1	M_1	NA	5-HT$_1$	5-HT$_2$	5-HT$_3$	
Imipramine	-	-	+	+	+	+	0.1-4% *In overdose:* 3.8-8%
Paroxetine	o	o	o	I	+	+	Prolonged seizures during ECT *In overdose:* No seizures in 15 patients with maximum dose 850 mg
Sertraline	o	o	o	+	+	I	Rare reports of seizures secondary to SIADH *In overdose:* No seizures in 40 patients up to 8000 mg
Fluoxetine	o	o	o	+	+	+	<1/1000[a]
Citalopram	o	o	o	+	+	+	No worsening of epilepsy in 16 patients *In overdose:* 100 mg – 1.9 g: 18% seizures; >1.9g: 49% seizures
Reboxetine	o	o/-	+	o	o	o	0.13%[a]
Venlafaxine	o	o	+	+	+	+	0.18%[a] *In overdose:* Seizures in dosages over 1000 mg
Nefazodone	o	o	o	+	-	+	No seizures in pre-marketing trials, since then rare reports of convulsions[a]
Mirtazapine	-	o	+	+	-	-	<0.1%[a]

Notes:
0, no/negligible effect; +, stimulation; -, blockade; [a]information from pre-marketing trials and product monograph. Receptors: H_1, histamine; M_1, muscarinic; NA, noradrenaline; 5-HT$_1$, 5-HT$_2$, 5-HT$_3$, serotonin. SIADH = Increased antidiuretic hormone secretion.

The latest generation of antidepressants has been developed to derive their therapeutic benefits from tailor-made action at specific monoamine receptors and re-uptake sites, in theory provoking better efficacy and better tolerability (Feighner, 1999).

Reboxetine is a selective noradrenergic re-uptake inhibitor (NARI) with low affinity for histaminergic, cholinergic, dopaminergic and alpha 1 adrenergic receptors. It appears to be equally effective to the tricyclics in treating depression; there is a suggestion it may be more effective than fluoxetine (Montgomery, 1997).

Venlafaxine is a serotonin-noradrenergic re-uptake inhibitor (SNRI), which is similar to the earlier generation of antidepressants, but it does not interact with histaminergic or cholinergic receptors, thus diminishing side effects due to those receptor systems. Several studies have indicated equipotentiability or superior antidepressant effectiveness with this compound compared to tricyclics. (Burnett and Dinan, 1994).

Nefazodone is a noradrenaline-serotonin re-uptake inhibitor, the most potent action of which is blockade of $5HT_2$ post-synaptic receptors, leading to a dual mechanism of action on the serotonin system. Noradrenaline re-uptake inhibition is only minimal, and there is no interaction with histamine or cholinergic receptors.

Mirtazapine, (a NASSA), has a selective action at alpha 2 adrenoreceptors, and only at some serotonin receptor subtypes. Its actions are to increase noradrenergic and serotonergic transmission by blocking the alpha 2 autoreceptors. However, because it also blocks $5HT_2$ and $5HT_3$ receptors, the increased serotonin turnover only stimulates the $5HT_1$ receptors. Thus it enhances noradrenergic and $5HT_{1A}$ -mediated serotonergic neurotransmission. It is free from muscarinic, alpha 1 adrenergic, and $5HT_2$ and $5HT_3$ related side effects, but its effect on histamine receptors can cause sedation and increased appetite. Several studies have shown equal or superior efficiency of this compound compared to other antidepressants (Bremner, 1995).

New antidepressant drugs and seizures

With regards to a broader spectrum of behaviours, there are over 30 studies of the use of SSRIs in the management of perseverative behaviour in patients with learning disability, including the spectrum of obsessive compulsive behaviours. However, the studies were largely uncontrolled, although the reports suggest that an improvement of behaviour can occur with relatively low doses. (Aman et al.,1999).

All of the SSRIs have been associated with seizures in clinical practice, although there is some evidence which suggests that they may have less seizure potential than the earlier agents.

Krijzer *et al.*, (1984) used freely moving rats implanted with subcortical electrodes. Almost all of the antidepressants tested caused epileptogenic EEG changes, with mianserin being the most potent. However, fluvoxamine caused only minimal effects.

None of the newer agents have been tested in such models and clinical information is largely derived from the clinical trials and post-marketing surveys. Generally the figures for seizure incidence given for all of these new compounds are less than for the tricyclic antidepressants, the lowest figures being recorded so far for mirtazapine and nefazodone.

Citalopram has been used in depression in patients with epilepsy. No change of seizure frequency was noted in 16 patients in an open study (Specchio *et al.*, 1997). In another study, Hovorka *et al.*, (2000) gave citalopram to 43 patients with epilepsy and co-morbid depression, and assessed them over an eight-week period. Sixty five percent were judged to be responders to the antidepressant effect. No change in seizure frequency was noted, and no de novo generalised tonic-clonic seizures were observed.

The SSRI most used in patients with epilepsy is paroxetine. Blumer (1997) has reported on the effective use of this drug in the management of patients with what he refers to as the inter-ictal dysphoric disorder of epilepsy. In his studies, paroxetine is often given in combination with a tricyclic antidepressant. He reports this combination to be safe and efficacious in this population. Exacerbation of seizures was not reported, and dysphoric symptoms resolved in the majority of his cases.

We have observed three patients with persistent epilepsy who have become seizure-free on paroxetine. In one, the effect was short-lived, but in the other two the effect has been sustained, in spite of no changes to the anticonvulsant prescriptions.

The other SSRI recently evaluated in epilepsy is sertraline (Kanner *et al.*, 2000). These investigators evaluated prospectively the effect of this antidepressant in 100 consecutive patients with epilepsy and depression (n−97) or obsessive compulsive disorder (n=3). They noted an increase in seizures following the start of therapy in 6% of patients, assessed from 0.2 to 38 months. Interestingly, the mean dose of sertraline in these patients was lower than in the other patients. They reported that the depressive symptoms resolved in 54% of patients, but noted the pleomorphic clinical picture of these patients, as described by Blumer (1997), and the symptom differences from typical major affective disorder.

Pharmacokinetic interactions

It has been emphasised for a long time now that serum anticonvulsant level monitoring can be of value in obtaining good seizure control, and checking compliance. The administration of additional drugs can cause metabolic interactions, leading to either a fall or a rise in the anticonvulsant serum levels. This may lead to a recrudescence or a worsening of seizure frequency, or precipitate anticonvulsant toxicity.

There are occasional but nevertheless important reports of interactions between tricyclic antidepressant drugs and both phenytoin and carbamazepine, leading to intoxication. The case of viloxazine has also been noted above.

The new generation of antidepressant drugs differs considerably in its ability to induce liver enzymes of the P450 system. Most psychotropic drugs are metabolised by four isoenzymes (CYP1A2, CYP2C, CYP2D6 and CYP3A4) (Monaco and Cicolin, 1999). The anticonvulsants mainly affect CYP3A4, and thus there is some potential for pharmacokinetic interactions.

In general, drugs which induce liver enzymes may lower the levels of antidepressant drugs, and this may have therapeutic consequences. Information on the effect of SSRIs on plasma levels of anticonvulsants is limited, although there are reports of carbamazepine toxicity in patients given fluoxetine (Dursun et al., 1993). Keller et al., (1997) looked for interactions between fluoxetine and carbamazepine in patients with epilepsy, but did not notice any change of plasma levels over an observation period of 20 days. Fluoxetine has also been associated with case histories of increased phenytoin (Jalil, 1992) and sodium valproate levels (Cruz-Flores et al., 1995).

Sertraline has less of an influence on concomitant anticonvulsant levels, probably because it has little or no effect on the cytochrome P450 3A4 system. However, possible interactions between sertraline and lamotrigine have been suggested (Kaufman and Gerner, 1998).

Paroxetine also does not inhibit the CYP3A4 system, and may not therefore provoke any interactions. The limited clinical data on 20 patients with epilepsy given this drug did not reveal any significant alteration of anticonvulsant levels (Data on file – GlaxoSmithKline).

With regards to the newer non-SSRI agents, no information is available.

ON THE USE OF ANTIDEPRESSANTS IN PATIENTS WITH LEARNING DISABILITY

As noted, there are very few specific studies in this area. The main data relate to SSRIs, and do not specifically address epilepsy. Since mood disorders in the learning-disabled population are often atypical, chronic and sometimes rapid-cycling, and as mood disorder in epilepsy is also atypical (for example, often taking the pattern of the inter-ictal dysphoric disorder), diagnostic issues are complicated, which makes treatment issues even more difficult.

Certainly to prescribe antidepressants without good clinical grounds in this population is to be discouraged. However, some studies have noted improvements in possible depression-related symptoms such as aggression and self injury, even with the presence of autism, but the development of treatment-emergent effects must be carefully sought, and this includes the onset of hypomanic-type symptoms, which in a study of fluoxetine occurred in 25% of the index population (Cook *et al.*, 1992).

Conclusions

The data with regards to the use of antidepressants in epilepsy suggest that nearly all of the tricyclic antidepressant drugs are proconvulsant, but there are clinical reports that, at least with some of them, an anticonvulsant effect has been noted. The reasons for this paradoxical effect are unclear.

In psychiatric practice, in recent years, there has been a move away from the use of tricyclic drugs, mainly on account of their other side effects and risk of death with overdose. In patients with a reduced seizure threshold, though not necessarily having a diagnosis of epilepsy, they should be avoided. Other drugs that are proconvulsant include maprotiline and mianserin.

Of the newer generation of drugs, the SSRIs appear to provoke less in the way of seizures than the tricyclic drugs. It is a possibility that the even newer, more selective drugs provoke less in the way of seizures than the SSRIs, but more data on these compounds are needed.

Metabolic interactions occur with some of these compounds, which may lead to anticonvulsant toxicity. Any change in symptoms reported by patients, or a deterioration of the affective disorder, that may suggest intoxication, should be sought. Whichever drug is used, it is advisable to start with smaller doses, if clinical needs allow, and increase the dose relatively slowly in order to avoid precipitation of potential seizures.

Data from people with learning disability are scarce, and clinical trials are urgently needed.

ANTIPSYCHOTIC DRUGS

A classification of the antipsychotic drugs is given in Table 5. As with antidepressant drugs, in recent years there have been several newer agents introduced into clinical practice. With some exceptions, these fall into the class of atypical antipsychotics.

Table 6 gives a review of the receptor binding profiles of a number of these agents.

The classic neuroleptic drugs, such as chlorpromazine and haloperidol, antagonise dopamine D_2 receptors. Essentially their clinical efficiency has been shown to correlate with inhibitory activity at these receptor subtypes. However, these

Table 5.   Antipsychotic drugs

Phenothiazines
Butyrophenones
Atypical
Others (sulpiride; tetrabenazine)

Table 6.   Receptor binding profiles of antipsychotics

Drug	Affinity for receptor (K_i in nmol/l)								
	D_1	D_2	D_4	α_1	α_2	H_1	$5\text{-}HT_{2a}$	$5\text{-}HT_{2c}$	M
Haloperidol	25	1	5	46	360	>1000	78	>1000	570
Clozapine	85	126	9	7	8	6	12	8	1.0
Risperidone	75	3	7	2	3	155	0.6	26	>1000
Olanzapine	31	112	27	19	228	7	4	11	2.1
Quetiapine	455	160	NA	7	87	11	220	615	56

Notes:
Receptors: D_1, D_2, D_4, dopamine; α_1, α_2, adrenergic; M, muscarinic; $5\text{-}HT_{2a}$, $5\text{-}HT_{2c}$, serotonin; H_1, histamine; NA, not available.
Source: Information from pre-marketing trials and product monographs.

drugs block dopamine receptors in the striatum leading to catalepsy in animal models, and unwanted extrapyramidal side effects in clinical practice.

The new generation of antipsychotic drugs fall into two categories; those that are clozapine related, including olanzapine and quetiapine, and others such as risperidone, sertindole and amisulpride.

Although clozapine has been available for many years, it was initially removed from clinical practice (except in some selected countries) on account of its potential to produce agranulocytosis. However, it was reintroduced as a model of an atypical antipsychotic.

Thus, the term relates to the low potential of these compounds to cause extrapyramidal problems; they also have minimal effects on serum prolactin levels. The mechanism of their atypicality seems to relate to different receptor profiles.

In general, the atypical antipsychotics occupy lower levels of D_2 receptors than the classical antipsychotics (20 – 60 % as opposed to 80 – 90%) (Kapur *et al.*, 1999). One reason for the profile of these agents may be due to their rapid displacement from receptors by endogenous dopamine, since they are more loosely bound.

The newer antipsychotic agents also have a lower relative affinity for striatal D_2 receptors as opposed to limbic D_2 receptors (dorsal –v- ventral striatum). Further, of all the newer agents, clozapine is the one that seems not to bind to the core of the nucleus accumbens.

Ever since their introduction, antipsychotic drugs have been shown to be proconvulsant. Early animal models, using the photosensitive baboon *Papio papio*, suggested that there may be differences between the phenothiazine-derived agents, such as chlorpromazine, and the butyrophenones, represented for example by haloperidol and pimozide.

Pimozide in particular seemed to have less effect on the seizure threshold. In clinical practice this drug has recently been problematic to prescribe because of the need to carry out electrocardiographic investigations before prescription. It is one of a growing number of drugs associated with prolongation the Q-T interval, with the possibility of being associated with cardiac complications.

In general, the use of intramuscular preparations, such as fluphenazine decanoate, was not associated with any change in the frequency of reporting of seizures in patients with epilepsy who also have psychosis.

As with the newer antidepressants, there is much less information about the effect of the atypical neuroleptics on the seizure threshold, with the single exception of clozapine. The latter was known to be proconvulsant from early studies, the seizures resulting from a dose-related effect. The incidence of seizures rises to about 5% at doses of 600mg, although EEG changes may be recorded at lower doses. The seizures are often myoclonic, but can be generalised tonic-clonic, or partial, depending on the individual patient.

It is perhaps no coincidence that the drug which appears to be the most effective antipsychotic, namely clozapine, is also associated with a high frequency of seizures.

The relationship of convulsive seizures to the relief of psychopathology is an integral part of psychiatric therapy, through ECT. It is often forgotten that the latter was introduced for the treatment of dementia praecox, and has clinically and theoretically important antipsychotic effects.

There are some patients with epilepsy who are non-responsive to neuroleptic drugs, and need clozapine. In particular there is a group of patients whose seizure frequency decreases or who become seizure-free, whose psychosis deteriorates in this setting. For them clozapine may be the drug of choice.

Case history

A 30-year-old patient, diagnosed as having leucine-sensitive hypoglycaemia at 10 months of age developed epilepsy at the age of four years. This typically presented with clusters of several episodes daily, lasting three or four days, recurring at monthly intervals. During her seizure she would have a typical aura with a feeling of fear and butterflies in her stomach lasting about 30 seconds. This was followed by a scream, and a generalised seizure, which would last about a minute. Prior to these seizures she would often have a prodrome of 2 – 3 days with a build up of verbal and physical aggression.

She had been treated with various medications, but at the age of 26 she was changed to sodium valproate, and her seizure frequency improved; indeed she became seizure-free. She had gradually developed a psychotic illness, but this dramatically deteriorated with resolution of the seizures and, aged 26 and 27, she was admitted twice to psychiatric hospitals under the Mental Health Act.

An EEG had revealed left anterior temporal abnormalities, and an MRI scan showed prominent ventricles.

She had been prescribed several antipsychotic drugs, including the atypical antipsychotics risperidone and olanzapine. None of these were of any help in resolving her psychosis. She was therefore started on clozapine, in gradually increasing doses. Her EEG was initially monitored.

On clozapine, her EEG revealed more frequent sharp waves over the left temporal region, and she began to develop auras again, although she had no complex partial or generalised seizures. The auras were simple partial attacks, and were of little concern to her.

A dramatic improvement in her psychosis was noted, such that she is once again living independently in the community, with stable mood, infrequent auditory hallucinations, and with more insight into her paranoia. She remains on sodium valproate, and clozapine (400 mg a day).

Reporting rates for the incidence of seizures with the other atypical antipsychotics vary from 0.1% in double-blind clinical trials of risperidone, to 0.2 – 0.9% for olanzapine, and 9 out of 1,710 cases for quetiapine. These figures come from the reporting of seizures in clinical trials, and do not necessarily reflect a causal relationship between prescription of the drug and the seizure event.

Pharmacokinetic interactions

The interactions between antipsychotic drugs and antiepileptic drugs have been even less studied than the antidepressants. Whilst some psychotropics, such as haloperidol, are mainly metabolised using the P450 system, others such as chlorpromazine use different liver enzyme systems. However, decreases in some neuroleptics can occur in patients prescribed anticonvulsant drugs, and several studies have been carried out in patients with schizophrenia who have received both carbamazepine and a neuroleptic.

Haloperidol levels can drop by up to 50% following co-administration of the antiepileptic (Arana *et al.*, 1986). Clozapine and olanzapine primarily use the CYP1A2 isoenzyme, which may lead to interactions with some of the tricyclic antidepressants and carbamazepine.

Antipsychotic use in patients with learning disability

As with the antidepressants, the studies carried out are largely anecdotal and of open design, although more recently, in the non-epileptic population, a number of atypical antipsychotic drugs have been used in a more controlled fashion (Aman and Madrid, 1999). In general, atypical antipsychotics are preferred in this population, not least for their potential effect on negative symptoms, and because of the reduced risk of the development of tardive motor abnormalities.

The majority of data published has been with clozapine and risperidone and most studies have suggested improved behaviour, relating not only to the psychosis, but also to reduced self-injury. Two studies in this area have been double-blind and both have been with risperidone (McDougle et al., 1995; Conduct Study Group, 1999). Both studies (using 1-6mg per day) reported significant improvements in a variety of target behaviours, although this did not appear to be diagnosis specific. Sedation and weight gain were the main problems.

Conclusions

As with antidepressants, further work needs to be done with antipsychotic agents in the important area of managing patients with learning disability and co-morbid epilepsy.

At the time of writing, particularly in epilepsy, the tendency is away from using the more traditional neuroleptics, to using the atypical neuroleptics for several reasons. The main one relates to the potential danger of the long-term development of extrapyramidal motor disorders, which are much less likely to occur with the atypical neuroleptics. These drugs are mainly well-tolerated by patients with epilepsy, and seizures are not usually a problem clinically.

Clozapine can be used in patients with epilepsy, particularly if the psychosis is proving intractable to treatment. We introduce the drug slowly, and monitor the EEG. We warn patients that their seizure frequency may rise. However, at doses below about 600mg/day, we have not encountered clinical problems. One particular caution relates to the development of the agranulocytosis, and patients (in the UK at least) need to be placed on a special register, and also have regular haematological assessments. Further, it is a contraindication to prescribe clozapine at the same time as carbamazepine.

OTHER PSYCHOTROPIC AGENTS

Patients with epilepsy are prescribed a variety of other psychotropic medications, the main ones being benzodiazepines, either as hypnotics or anticonvulsants, and lithium, a mood stabiliser.

Benzodiazepines should be used with caution in patients with epilepsy, the main problem being the potential for a paradoxical increase in seizures, or withdrawal seizures on stopping the drug. Further, some of these drugs have a potential for the development of dependency.

There appear to be differences between the 1,5- and 1,4-benzodiazepines, the former represented by clobazam. This drug was introduced initially as an anxiolytic, but was shown to have effective and sustained anticonvulsant properties. It is recommended as an adjunct treatment for the management of patients with intractable epilepsy, and may be particularly of value in patients with epilepsy with a high level of anxiety, who may also present with panic attacks. It is less cerebrotoxic than the 1,4-benzodiazepines such as clonazepam, and is recognised to have inherent psychotropic properties.

Clobazam is of particular value in patients with intermittent clusters of seizures (such as catamenial episodes), and for the suppression of clusters of seizures. The latter are associated in some patients with post-ictal psychosis, and prevention of the cluster may well abort a potential psychosis.

These post-ictal behaviour changes can be quite subtle, but nevertheless very disruptive in the learning-disabled. Close observation is required for their detection, and the link between the seizures and the behaviour changes are not always clear. Thus, the well-established lucid interval can be quite confusing. This is a period of 'normal' behaviour which follows the seizures, and may be as long as 24-48 hours, before the post-ictal behaviour changes often suddenly erupt. These behaviour changes may be psychotic, but are often more of the irritable, dysphoric and aggressive pattern.

These can be well-controlled by the judicious use of clobazam, and 10mg given 4-6 hourly for 24-48 hours may be all that is required. Clobazam can also be given after the seizure cluster, if any psychiatric symptoms seem to be developing, using a similar dosage schedule.

In general, anxiolytic drugs, particularly of the benzodiazepine variety, are not advocated for the control of behaviour in patients with learning disability, and there are no studies from which to guide treatment (Werry, 1998). The same essentially can be said about the use of beta- blockers in this population. They have been used more for the management of aggression than anxiety, although their use in managing tremor may also occasionally be warranted (Ruedrich and Erhardt, 1999).

Lithium, which is also proconvulsant, can be used as a mood-stabiliser in patients who have recurrent cyclical mood disorders, or recurrent outbursts of affective aggressive behaviors. Caution should be exercised when combining lithium with carbamazepine, since patients occasionally develop a cerebrotoxic syndrome. Monitoring of serum levels of lithium is mandatory, as is observing patients over time for the development of secondary complications of lithium therapy such as hypothyroidism, or diabetes insipidus.

Small double-blind trials of lithium in patients with learning disability have been performed showing reduction of mood-cycling (Rivinus and Harmatz, 1979). However, the development of side effects may well be more problematic in this population, particularly tremor and incontinence. Further, recognition of signs of lithium-induced central nervous system toxicity may be more difficult. Clearly monitoring of serum levels is crucial.

There is a case for the use of some psycho-stimulants, particularly in the management of attention deficit hyperactivity disorder. The group of drugs used mainly is the amphetamines and related drugs, for example methylphenidate. In the past, these medications were sometimes prescribed to people with severe epilepsy to counteract the sedative effect of the anticonvulsants, but this can no longer be advocated. The effects of these drugs, particularly methylphenidate, on the seizure threshold is not clear, and the value of these compounds in patients with epilepsy and learning disability has not been studied (Zagnoni and Albano, 2002).

CONCLUSIONS

Psychotropic drugs are used with considerable frequency in patients with epilepsy, and used appropriately and cautiously they add considerably to management. However, like all CNS-active drugs, they have a variety of side effects, and the exacerbation or precipitation of seizures is important in this patient group. It is particularly relevant in patients who may have been seizure-free for a period of time, and who then go on to develop psychiatric disorders.

There has been an expansion in the number of psychotropic drugs available in recent years, particularly with regards to the antidepressants and the antipsychotics. The newly developed agents generally seem to have a more favourable profile than older agents for use in patients with epilepsy.

Patients with learning disability and epilepsy would seem to be particularly vulnerable to the development of behaviour disorders and the prescription of psychotropic drugs in this population is considerable. It is important that physicians have an intricate knowledge of the mechanisms of action and most appropriate prescription doses and titration schedules of these drugs, but also to have an awareness of their side effects. The latter may be particularly prevalent, and are often difficult to discern in patients with learning disability.

The problems of exacerbating epilepsy are ever-present, although an awareness of the opposite, namely a deterioration of behaviour when epilepsy improves, also requires considerable thought, and is certainly one indication for the careful choice of a psychotropic agent. Further studies in this area are clearly needed.

REFERENCES

Aman, M. G., Arnold, L. E. and Armstrong, S. E. (1999). *Ment Retard Dev Disabil Res Rev* **5**, 279-289.

Aman, M.G. and Madrid, S. (1999). Atypical antipsychotics in persons with developmental disabilities. *Ment Retard Dev Disabil Res Rev* **5**, 253-263.

Arana, G. W., Goff, D. C., Freidman, H. *et al.* (1986). Does carbamazepine induced reduction in haloperidol plasma levels worsen psychotic symptoms? *Am J Psychiatry* **143**, 658-659.

Blumer, D. (1997). Antidepressant and double antidepressant treatment for the affective disorder of epilepsy. *J Clin Psychiatry* **58**, 3-11.

Bremner, J. D. (1995). A double blind comparison of ORG 3770, amitriptyline and placebo in major depression. *J Clin Psychiatry* **57**, 519-526.

Burley, D. M. (1977). A brief note on the problem of epilepsy and antidepressant treatment. In: Jewkes, A (Ed), *Depression; the Biochemical and Physiological Role of Ludiomil.* Ciba, Horsham, pp 202-203.

Burnett, F. E. and Dinan, T. G. (1994). The clinical effectiveness of venlafaxine in the treatment of depression. *Reviews of Contemporary Pharmacotherapy* **9**, 303-320.

Conduct Study Group (October 1999). Multisite study of risperidone versus placebo in children with sub-average IQs and comorbid conduct disorder. Oppositional Defiant Disorder or Conduct Disorder NOS. Quoted by Aman and Madrid 1999.

Cook, E. H., Rowlett, R., Jaselskis, C. *et al.* (1992). Fluoxetine treatment of children and adults with autistic disorder and mental retardation. *J Am Acad Child Adolesc Psychiatry* **31**, 739-745.

Cruz-Flores, S., Ghazala, R., Hyat, R. and Mirza, W. (1995). Valproate toxicity with fluoxetine therapy. *Missouri medicine* **92**, 296-297.

Dursun, S. M., Mathew, V. M. and Reveley, M. A. (1993). Toxic serotonin syndrome after fluoexetine plus carbamazepine. *Lancet* **342**, 442-443.

Edwards, J. G. and Glen-Bott, M. (1984). Does viloxazine have epileptogenic properties. *J Neurol Neurosurg Psychiatry* **47**, 960 – 964.

Edwards, J. G. (1985). Antidepressants and seizures: epidemiological and clinical aspects. In: Trimble M.R. (Ed), *The Psychopharmacology of Epilepsy.* J Wiley & Sons, Chichester, pp 119-139.

Feighner, G. P. (1999). Mechanism of action of antidepressant medication. J *Clin Psychiatry* **60**, 4-11.

Garvey, M. J. and Tollefson, G. D. (1987). Occurrence of myoclonus in patients treated with cyclic antidepressants. *Arch Gen Psychiatry* **44**, 269 – 272.

Hovorka, J., Herman, E. and Nemcova, I. (2000). Treatment of interictal depression with citalopram in patients with epilepsy. *Epilepsy and Behaviour* **6**, 444-448.

Jalil, P. (1992). Toxic reaction following the combined administration of fluoxetine and phenytoin. *J Neurol Neurosurg Psychiatry* **55**, 412-413.

Jick, H., Dinan, B. J., Hunter, J. R. *et al.* (1983). Tricyclic antidepressants and convulsions. *J Clin Psychopharmacol* **3**, 182-185.

Kanner, A.M., Kozak, A.M. and Frey, M. (2000). The use of sertraline in patients with epilepsy, is it safe? *Epilepsy and Behaviour* **1**, 100-105.

Kapur, S., Zipursky, R. B. and Remmington, G. (1999). Clinical and theorectical implications of 5HT$_2$ and D$_2$ receptor occupancy of clozapine, risperidone and alanzapine. *Am J Psychiatry* **156**, 286-293.

Kaufman, K. R. and Gerner, R. (1998). Lamotrigine toxicity secondary to sertraline. *Seizure* **7**, 163-165.

Keller, R., Tortar Prolo, P., Ravizza, L. and, Monaco, F. (1997). Interazioni Farmacocinetiche Tra Fluoxetina e Farmaci anti epilettici. *Bolletino Lega Italiana Contro L'epilepsia* **99**, 183-186.

Krijzer, F., Snelder, M. and Bradford, D. (1984). Comparison of the proconvulsant properties of fluvoxamine and clovoxamine with either other antidepressants in an animal model. *Neuropsychobiology* **12**, 249-254.

Krishnamoorthy, E. S. and Trimble, M.R. (2002). Neuropsychiatric disorders in epilepsy – epidemiology and classification. In: Trimble, M.R. and Schmitz, B. (Eds), *The Neuropsychiatry of Epilepsy*. Cambridge University Press, Cambridge, pp. 5-17.

Luchins, D. J., Oliver, A. P. and Wyatt, R. J. (1984). Seizures with antidepressants: an in vitro technique to assess relative risk. *Epilepsia* **25**, 25-32.

McDougle, C. J., Brodkin, E. S., Yeung, P.P. *et al.* (1995). Risperidone in adults with autism or pervasive developmental disorder. *J Child Adolesc Psychopharmacol* **5**, 273-282.

Meldrum, B. S., Anlezark, G., Adam, H. K. and Greenwood, D. T. (1982). Anticonvulsant and proconvulsant properties and viloxazine hydrochloride. *Psychopharmacology* **76**, 212-217.

Monaco, F. and Cicolin, A. (1999). Interactions between anticonvulsants and psychoactive drugs. *Epilepsia* **40**, S71 – S76.

Montgomery, S. A. (1997). Reboxetine: additional benefits to depressed patients. *J Psychopharmacol* **11** (Suppl), S9-S15.

Noble, S. and Benfield, P. (1997). Citalopram: a review of its pharmacology, clinical efficiency and tolerability in the treatment of depression. *CNS Drugs* **8**, 410-431.

Ojemann, L. M., Friel, P. N., Trejow, J. and Dudley, D. L (1983). Effect of doxepin on seizure frequency and depressed epileptic patients. *Neurology* **33**, 646 – 648.

Pisani, F., Narvone, M. C., Fazio, A. *et al.* (1984). Increased serum carbamazepine levels by viloxazine in epileptic patients. *Epilepsia* **25**, 482-485.

Rivinus, R. and Harmatz, J. (1979). Diagnosis and lithium treatment of affective disorder in the retarded: 5 case studies. *Am J Psychiatry* **36**, 551-554.

Ruedrich, S.L. and Erhardt, D. (1999). Beta adrenergic blockers in mental retardation and mental disabilities. *Ment Retardation Ment Disabil Res Rev* **5**, 290-298.

Sachdev, P. S. (1992). Psychoactive drug use in an institution for intellectually handicapped persons. *Med J Australia* **155**, 75-79.

Specchio, L. M., La Neve, A., Spinelli, A. et al. (1997). Il trattamento antidepressevo con Citalopram in pazienti con epilessia. *Bolletino Lega Italiana Crontro L'epilessia* **99**, 187-188.

Trimble, M. R. (1980). New antidepressant drugs and the seizure threshold, *Neuropharmacology*, **19**, 1127 – 1128.

Trimble, M. R. (1987). Antidepressant drugs seizures and epilepsy. *Quo Vadis*, Publication of the Sanofi Group, Montpellier.

Trimble, M. R., Anlezark, G. and Meldrum, B. (1977). Seizure activity in photosensitive baboons following antidepressant drugs, and the role of serotoninergic mechanisms. *Psychopharmacology* **51**, 159-164.

Werry, J. S. (1998). Anxiolytics. In: Reiss, S. and Aman, M. G. (Eds), *Psychotropic Medications and Developmental Disabilities: the International Consensus Handbook*. Nisongir Center OSU, Columbus, Ohio pp201-214.

Zagnoni, P. G. and Albano, C. (2002). Psychostimulants in epilepsy. *Epilepsia* **43** (Suppl 2), 28-31.

Learning Disability and Epilepsy: an Integrative Approach
Edited by Michael R. Trimble
© 2003 Clarius Press Ltd

11

Non-Medical Interventions for People with Epilepsy and Learning Disability

TIM BETTS, KATIE GOULD AND LYN GREENHILL

Birmingham University Seizure Clinic
Queen Elizabeth Psychiatric Hospital
Birmingham, UK

INTRODUCTION

Before considering specific non medical treatments for people with epilepsy who have learning disability, a few general words are indicated. People with learning disability are particularly likely to have epilepsy. This may be syndromic or it may be a reflection of general brain disturbance. People with mild learning disability are perhaps four to five times more likely to have epilepsy than their non-affected peer group and up to 50% of people with severe learning disability will have concomitant epilepsy. This is usually thought to be due to whatever it is that is causing the learning disability rather than being a direct relationship between the two conditions (although there are possible exceptions to this).

People with learning disability are usually excluded from clinical trials of new anticonvulsant drugs and, even if they are included or a specific trial done, special considerations regarding consent often limit the strength of the trial, and authors of the trial may be so intent on getting some kind of result from it that they can potentially stretch results further than they should (Crawford *et al.*, 2001). In a recent review of clinical trials of anti-epileptic drugs in people with learning disability and epilepsy it was shown that, despite the prevalence of epilepsy in people with learning difficulty, there are very few anti-epileptic trials and most not of the standard that we have come to expect (Working Group of the International Association for the Scientific

Study of Intellectual Disability, 2001). That paper also outlined in some detail the care context of people with epilepsy who also have learning disability. It showed that for people with learning disability and epilepsy, assessing the impact of epilepsy goes far beyond merely assessing the impact of the seizures or the drugs themselves. This of course has become increasingly clear in epilepsy in general. Several recent papers have shown that, whether or not the child or adult has learning disability, care consists of much more than just trying to control seizures with drugs, and the impact of the epilepsy is not just on the person that has it, but also on friends, relatives and supporters (Brown et al., 1998; Hayden *et al.*, 1992; Ellis *et al.*, 2000; Verma & Nichols, 1993; Espie *et al.*, 1999).

In learning disability these stresses on the family members may be extreme and long-lasting and may to some extent influence the family's approach to new treatments, particularly if they seem potentially hazardous (Farnalls and Renwick, 2003).

In days gone by, in the UK and elsewhere, people with intellectual disability, perhaps particularly if they had epilepsy, were shut away in institutions. Latterly an attempt has been made to draw them out of institutions (the old subnormality hospitals) into the community either to live in group homes or with their parents and supporters. This has the advantage of making them more visible but at the same time what expertise there had been developed in subnormality hospitals in regard to epilepsy does not always shift into the community where learning difficulty often becomes not so much the care of specialist epilepsy services but more the responsibility of general practitioners whose knowledge of epilepsy is often limited. It is into this breach, that the learning disability nurse has had to step and develop his or her knowledge of epilepsy, so that people with learning disability who also have epilepsy can obtain the investigations and care which they need but which, sadly, they often do not get.

Within the specialty of learning disability there are a few practitioners who take a particular interest in epilepsy. They are beginning to produce mission statements, care plans and ideas for the better and future management of people with learning disability who also happen to have epilepsy (Espie *et al.*, 1999; Kerr and Espie, 1997; Espie *et al.*, 1997). Even physicians with a conventional view of epilepsy are beginning to recognise that epilepsy and learning disability may be a challenge for the future (Hannah and Brodie, 1998).

Learning disability and epilepsy have three complications which can make the combination more difficult than epilepsy without learning disability. Firstly, learning the combination is not a single entity or a single syndrome. Secondly, people with learning disability may not get the investigations that they need or the best management of their epilepsy (Carvill *et al.*, 1999). Thirdly, there are diagnostic issues relating to epilepsy occurring in people with learning disability that are not found in the normal population (Paul, 1997). Since seizures in people with learning difficulty can be particularly difficult to distinguish from other forms of behaviour it is likely that the misdiagnosis rate in this population is particularly high.

Thus people with learning disability have epilepsy which may be hard to recognise or difficult to control, and they may respond differently and badly to conventional medication. Other methods of controlling seizures should, where possible, therefore be sought and conventional medication kept to a minimum. In this chapter we describe some of these.

RELAXATION

This general term applies to a variety of techniques which one uses to induce peaceful, relaxing thoughts in the mind and (usually) generalised relaxation of bodily muscles (occasionally specific to one or more groups). There is little doubt that general muscular relaxation (however it is achieved) can reduce seizure frequency both in adults and children. This is almost certainly true for people with learning disability. It is likely that for different people different and specific methods of relaxation are needed, but there is good scientific evidence that relaxation, both in adults and children, is good for people with epilepsy in general (there may be an exception in those people who need to maintain a high level of arousal to achieve and keep seizure freedom, but even they have to relax sometimes). The whole subject is well summarised by Dahl (1992). It is important to remember that some form of relaxation, even if not specifically mentioned as such as part of the treatment process, is common to many behavioural therapies and in a formal controlled trial must be allowed for in some way. In Schmid-Schönbein's illuminating study relaxation, even if not specifically sought, may have been part of what was a very successful behavioural treatment package (Schmid-Schönbein, 1998).

There are many ways of inducing relaxation. It is likely that most behavioural methods of treating epilepsy are more than relaxation, but it has to be proved that this is so. Most of the studies which attempt to tease out some of the variables and offer other treatment options in the non-medical treatment of epilepsy (for instance Schmid-Schönbein, 1998) are clearly dealing with people who do not have learning disability, but many of the treatments offered (perhaps with some adjustment to take account of learning difficulty) could be applied in this group of patients. Certainly Schmid-Schönbein's methods would have to be adapted to people with learning disability, but this would not be impossible to do, particularly if they were carried out by a person who knew the patient well.

BEHAVIOUR THERAPY AND EPILEPSY

There are many types of behaviour therapy and there have been several approaches to trying to use some aspects of behaviour therapy in managing epilepsy. Descriptions of two of the most successful ones can be found in the previously-mentioned paper of Schmid-Schönbein and the book by Dahl. Neither of them were describing behaviour therapy in people with learning disability as such but the principles are the same. Schmid-Schönbein first of all discussed the view (which has taxed the brains of many conventional therapists) whether one can recognise a form of epilepsy which is intractable from the beginning or whether, in fact, one has not tried hard enough to control seizures from the start. She then went on to describe techniques of self-control in a group of 16 patients with apparently intractable epilepsy of several years' standing. The techniques consisted of 'detailed self observation' which led to identifying warning signals of the beginning of a seizure, and seizure-provoking factors, and the development of 'counter measures (behavioural methods to interrupt the beginning of a seizure and to neutralise provoking factors)'. Many of the patients seemed to have strong psychic stress related to a seizure and poor intuitive self control abilities. It is likely that many people with epilepsy, learning-disabled or not, are like this. Those that achieved better control (68%) obtained a significant seizure reduction which seemed to be continued after the treatment ended.

To develop individual treatment strategies, there is necessarily prolonged continuity of care, which obviously takes a great deal of time and other confounding factors may have relevance to the treatment response. Dahl (1992) described a variety of behavioural techniques, including guided relaxation, to reduce anxiety about seizures, again with a significant degree of success. Both these techniques, if suitably modified and used in conjunction with a trained nurse, could be applied successfully to people with learning disability.

A variant of behaviour therapy, again with several variables, is practised by the Andrews / Reiter Epilepsy Research Programme in California (Andrews and Schonfield, 1992; Andrews et al., 2000; Andrews and Reiter, 2000). Their methods have developed over the years and carry a high success rate. Like other behavioural methods they depend on teaching the patient self control and the ability to recognise when a seizure is coming and to lower arousal as it does so, to identify pre-seizure warnings and to identify triggers to seizures. They report good results with behavioural treatment. It should be emphasised these are not usually in patients with learning disability, but with suitable modifications there is no reason why they should not be used in this group.

Behaviour therapies have several components to them. In a proper study of behaviour therapy to treat epilepsy it would be important to ensure that it was not just one aspect of the behaviour therapy (which almost always includes relaxation) which was responsible for the success. Furthermore, although the behaviour therapy may have a general input in every patient, it tends to be tailored to a particular individual in a way that drug therapy, apart from dosage, is not. Interestingly it is dosage which often changes when a drug actually gets onto the market, having undergone formal clinical trials!

Unless such factors are allowed for in assessing results, particularly in a double blind trial (with the assessors of the trial results totally removed from those who are conducting the therapy), then such a trial can look weak, to those who are more used to conventional medical double blind controlled trials. Any trial should separate the various aspects of therapy so that individual factors can be judged in isolation. This would be possible to do in epilepsy, but would require a large number of subjects and, since these techniques do not just involve offering a drug (which can be done by anybody), the requisite number of therapists. This is probably one of the reasons why trials in this area have rarely been performed although, if money was available, they could be. Learning difficulty could be one of the variables in such a trial, or assessed separately.

Many behaviour therapies involve the patient changing arousal very quickly once an oncoming seizure is identified. Some patients, if they detect a seizure (and detection of an oncoming seizure, even if untrained and not formally recognised, is commoner than we realise) can do this by increasing arousal and trying to develop a high degree of concentration. Although this may be initially successful, our own experience is that it is difficult to maintain this at a high level for very long and it may be better for most patients to lower arousal if they feel a seizure coming on. Since a seizure is frightening and disturbing, a warning of one, particularly if he or she feels powerless to stop it, may mean that arousal reduction is difficult, unless the process becomes automatic and the patient hardly has to think about it. Many apparently successful therapies with different methods may in fact be successful because they do, sometimes without the operator realising it, reduce stress and anxiety and therefore reduce arousal.

People with learning disability sometimes have problems in understanding verbal instructions. This need not be an insuperable handicap. Relaxation can be taught by other methods than verbal instruction and people with apparently no verbal communication can still be taught it, particularly by somebody who is well known to them and who they trust. Difficulty in communication in itself is not enough to deprive people from attempts at controlling seizures with behaviour therapy, although, as in people with normal intelligence, it would be important to try to establish the essential elements of the technique.

ACUPUNCTURE

There have been reports in the literature that acupuncture may have some effect in intractable epilepsy (reviewed in Kloster *et al.*, 1999). However these have been uncontrolled studies. Although experiments have suggested increased levels of endorphins in cerebrospinal fluid after electro-acupuncture and a significant increase in the cerebral content of opioids in rats after electro-acupuncture (Sonnen, 1997; Uhlmann and Froscher, 2001) both pro- and anti-convulsant actions of the body's natural opioid-peptides have been reported.

Kloster *et al.* (1999) used experienced Chinese acupuncturists and observers, who were unaware of whether treatment (electro-acupuncture) was active or control (inert electro-acupuncture - using sham points), in a well-designed controlled study, albeit with chronic patients and low patient and control numbers. The two treatments were no different in their effect; both produced a modest reduction in seizures, but only the placebo treatment produced a significant increase in the number of seizure-free weeks. The authors concluded that they had not been able to prove the beneficial effect of acupuncture in chronic intractable epilepsy. Obviously a better effect might occur in patients with new-onset seizures or less intractable epilepsy, but there was no effect in those patients most likely to be exposed to the treatment. This is in accordance with the views of Sonnen (1997) who in a long and somewhat sceptical chapter on the effect of alternative and folk remedies in epilepsy also found no evidence that acupuncture was effective

BIOFEEDBACK

Biofeedback (embracing different treatments, but all implying modification by the patient of a biological signal relating to the parameter to be changed) has had some exposure in epilepsy. Early studies in the 1970s suggested that it might be useful, but it was difficult to control learning effects which tended to disappear as soon as the treatment was stopped. Our own experiments with this treatment were abandoned. Latterly interest has been re-aroused in this method particularly in Germany (Uhlmann and Froscher, 2001). The interesting thing about the modern methods of biofeedback for epilepsy is that it is used not just to develop control over seizures but to treat mood as well (although it is difficult to say whether increasing a feeling of control over seizures lifts mood or vice versa). In the method advocated by Uhlmann and Froscher (2001) the apparatus used is rather complex (which the authors feel may add to the therapeutic value of the treatment). Wolf (1997) also favours biofeedback for some patients. Some have used it for seizure arrest in response to an aura (Caspers and Speckmann, 1969). This may be more suitable for people with learning difficulty. It could be argued that relaxation is not involved in biofeedback treatment, but at least in a modified sense it probably is and with renewed interest in it, particularly in Germany, it may be a behavioural treatment of the future although, like all behavioural treatments, it needs more scientific validation.

SEIZURE-ALERT DOGS

Some dogs seem to recognise that a particular patient's seizure is coming on before human companions, or the patient, themselves do (Brown and Strong, 2001). Untrained dogs can panic and become aggressive, but carefully trained dogs (trained with reward when a seizure occurs) can produce useful warnings of an oncoming seizure. A series of dogs have now been trained as companions to people with chronic epilepsy, both in this country and in America (Dalziel et al., 2003). Originally this was merely as support, so that they could get about more. An unexpected finding was that human subjects with epilepsy, given a trained seizure- alert dog, have a significant improvement in seizure rate (Brown and Strong, 2001). Seizure-alert dogs may therefore be very useful not only in helping people with intractable epilepsy to get out more but also in reducing their seizure frequency. Further research in this area is clearly needed.

HYPNOSIS

Hypnosis would appear to be a high arousal state of intense concentration as the person being hypnotised has to concentrate very hard on a particular body part or a particular sensation. Once they do this they appear to pass into a state of dissociation and suggestibility (although they remain completely aware of what is happening and retain control). By concentrating hard on a particular idea or feeling in this state of dissociation they may be able to accept suggestions about their future behaviour and automatically thereafter act on them (post-hypnotic suggestion). The technique can be used to help people directly abolish a seizure or to change their arousal if they feel one coming and there are some reports that in some individuals hypnosis may be effective (Betts and Greenhill, In Press).

It requires a degree of concentration on the part of the subject. Hypnosis also requires a hypnotist who is aware of the potential dangers of inducing a seizure in somebody with epilepsy and who, in particular, has learnt to avoid reminding the patient under the influence of hypnosis accidentally of situations that might induce a seizure. Waking up should be carried out slowly without a sudden change in arousal. In our experience people with epilepsy can be hypnotised as easily as people without epilepsy and, providing the hypnosis is done by somebody skilled, people with learning disability can be easily and reliably hypnotised. Hypnosis may be particularly useful with people that have seizures in particular situations or in particular frames of mind. Hypnosis can be adapted to people with learning difficulty. It is has not been systematically studied as much, but in isolated cases we have found it very helpful. 12% of subjects in one study completely lost their seizures using hypnosis alone (Efron, 1957).

AROMATHERAPY

This is a technique which involves a whole person massage with strongly smelling pleasant aromatic oils: in epilepsy usually a single oil is used. Massage with the oil reduces tension. The aim is to get the person to associate the smell of the particular oil used with the decrease in tension so that eventually merely smelling the oil will be enough to reduce tension instantly. Sometimes hypnosis is used to aid this conditioning. About a third of patients treated either with aromatherapy alone or aromatherapy and hypnosis achieve complete control of their seizures which appears to be relatively long-lasting (and continues for at least a year after the treatment stops) (Betts and Greenhill, In Press). Until fully controlled trials are carried out it is difficult to know what element of the treatment (or what combination of elements) is responsible for the success of this technique. Aromatherapy massage is very relaxing which may be one element of the treatment programme, but it does appear that those people who get most success from this treatment are those who develop a conditioned smell memory to the oil (Betts and Greenhill, In Press; Kirk-Smith et al., 1963). How much these results are a placebo effect cannot be determined from the current studies of the technique although it should be possible to develop a placebo controlled trial. Use of odour to control seizures has a long heritage (Betts and Betts, 1998).

OTHER REMEDIES

Sonnen (1997) commented 'even a silly looking theory can produce good results'. Medicine itself has successful treatments which clearly work (using the usual criteria for successful medical treatment) even though the theory about why these treatments work turns out to be totally wrong or is unavailable. So remedies such as folk treatments should not be ignored even though the theory behind them appears to be strange. Sonnen has reviewed many folk therapies for epilepsy and went to great length to try to produce evidence for them, but for most of the therapies there is no evidence or very little evidence that they might be effective in epilepsy and the studies are not controlled. One or two therapies would probably benefit from further more detailed studies and he rightly points out that in the developing world where expensive drugs are not available, alternative treatments that work reliably would be particularly helpful, although there is likely to be misconception about the illness and about its treatment.

Homeopathy is briefly mentioned with a choice of the particular agent depending more on the type of patient than on the particular type of epilepsy, but only a modest result is claimed in epilepsy even by the most enthusiastic supporters although formal testing in this matter has not been carried out (Sonnen, 1997).

There is a vast literature on herbal treatments for epilepsy and in some countries there is a long tradition of using them (Sonnen, 1997; Wolf, 1997). To some extent the agents depend on what plants are available in the country in which they are used, but it is interesting that the peony crops up in several formulae and was used in this country in Shakespeare's time (Betts, 1992). Some plant products have been shown to be potentially helpful in epilepsy, either by prolonging the half life of an anticonvulsant or by a direct effect on the person. Sonnen mentions several (interestingly again the peony amongst them) which would be worthy of further study.

In general terms the results of alternative and folk remedies are difficult to prove and often poor. Although most folk remedies are not dangerous, some can be and sudden withdrawal from anticonvulsant drugs if they are replaced by such treatments, even if they have previously appeared to be without effect, can be dangerous.

The growing interest in 'natural' remedies, even in the Western world, means that interest in these methods will continue. Some are promising and formal trials should be undertaken. The problem is that formal trials of compounds which are not drugs can be expensive and are difficult to finance.

CONCLUSION

In conclusion, non-medical treatments of epilepsy are not of proven value as yet, although there are certainly some methods which look promising. Some epilepsy experts, like Wolf and Betts are hopeful, others like Sonnen less sanguine. The time has surely come for formal trials of some of these methods that look promising.

REFERENCES

Andrews, S.D. and Reiter, J. (2000). A neurobehavioural approach for treatment of complex partial epilepsy: efficacy. *Seizure* **9**, 198-203.

Andrews, D., Reither, J., Schonfeld, W. *et al.* (2000). A neurobehavioural treatment for unilateral complex partial seizures: a comparison of right- and left-hemisphere patients. *Seizure* **9**, 189-197.

Andrews, D. and Schonfield, W. (1992). Predictive factors for controlling seizures using a behavioural approach. *Seizure* **1**, 111-116.

Betts, T. (1992). Epilepsy and stress. *Br Med J* **305**, 378-379.

Betts, T. and Betts, H. (1998). John Hall and his epileptic patients – epileptic management in early 17th century England. *Seizure* **7**, 411-414.

Betts, T. and Greenhill, L. Aromatherapy and hypnosis in the management of epilepsy. (chapter in press).

Brown, S., Betts, T., Crawford, C. *et al.* (1998). Epilepsy Needs Revisited: A revised epilepsy needs document for the UK. *Seizure* **7**, 435-446.

Brown, S. and Strong, V. (2001). The use of seizure-alert dogs. *Seizure* **10**, 39-41.

Carvill, S., Clarke, D. and Cassidy, G. (1999). The management of epilepsy in a hospital for people with a learning difficulty. *Seizure* **8**, 175-180

Caspers, H. and Speckmann, E-J. (1969). DC potential, shifts in paroxysmal states. In: Jasper, H., Ward, A., Pope, A. et al. (Eds), *Basic Mechanisms of the Epilepsies.* Little Brown, Boston, pp.375-388..

Crawford, P., Brown, S. and Kerr, M. (2001). A randomised open-label study of gabapentin and lamotrigine in adults with learning disability and resistant epilepsy. *Seizure* **10**, 107-115.

Dahl, J. (1992). *Epilepsy – a Behaviour Medicine Approach to Assessment and Treatment in Children.* Hogrefe and Huber, Seattle.

Dalziel, D., Uthman, B., McGorray, S. *et al.* (2003). Seizure-alert dogs: a review and preliminary study. *Seizure* **12**, 115-120.

Efron, R. (1957). The conditioned inhibition of uncinate fits. *Brain*, **80**, 251-252.

Ellis, N., Upton D. and Thompson, P. (2000). Epilepsy and the family: a review of current literature. *Seizure* **9**, 22-30.

Espie, C., Kerr, M., Paul, A. *et al.* (1997). Learning disability and epilepsy. 2. A review of available outcome measures and position statement on development priorities. *Seizure* **6**, 337-350.

Espie, C., Paul, A., McColl, J. *et al.* (1999). Cognitive functioning in people with epilepsy plus severe learning disabilities: a systematic analysis of predictors of daytime arousal and attention. *Seizure* **8**, 73-80.

Farnalls, S. and Renwick, J. (2003). Parents care giving approaches: facing a new treatment alternative in severe childhood epilepsy. *Seizure* **12**, 1-10.

Hannah, J. and Brodie, M. (1998). Epilepsy and learning disabilities – a challenge for the next millennium? *Seizure* **7**, 3-13.

Hayden, M., Penna, C. and Buchanan, N. (1992). Epilepsy: patient perceptions of their condition. *Seizure* **1**, 191-197.

Kerr, P. and Espie, C. (1997). Learning disability and epilepsy. 1. Towards common outcome measures. *Seizure* **6**, 331-336.

Kirk-Smith, M., Van Toller, C. and Dodd, G. (1963). Unconscious odour conditioning in human subjects. *Biol Psychiatry* **17**, 221-231.

Kloster, R., Larsson, P., Lossius, R. *et al.* (1999). The effect of acupuncture in chronic intractable epilepsy. *Seizure* **8**, 170-174.

Paul, A. (1997). Epilepsy or stereotypy? Diagnostic issues in learning disabilities. *Seizure* **6**, 111-120.

Schmid-Schönbein, C. (1998). Improvement of seizure control by psychological methods in patients with intractable epilepsies. *Seizure* **7**, 261-270.

Sonnen, A. (1997). Alternative and folk remedies. In: Engel, J. and Pedley, T. (Eds), *Epilepsy: a Comprehensive Textbook*. Lippincott-Raven, Philadelphia, pp.1365-1378.

Uhlmann, C. and Froscher, C. (2001). Biofeedback treatment in patients with refractory epilepsy: changes in depression and control orientation. *Seizure* **10**, 34-38.

Verma, N. and Nichols, C. (1993). Severity of neuropsychological function rather than etiology determines the severity of inter-ictal behaviour disorder. *Seizure* **2**, 105-109.

Wolf, P. (1997). Behavioral therapy. In: Engel, J. and Pedley, T. (Eds), *Epilepsy: A Comprehensive Textbook*. Lippincott-Raven, Philadelphia, pp.1359-1364.

Working Group of the International Association for the Scientific Study of Intellectual Disability (2001). Clinical guidelines for the management of epilepsy in adults with an intellectual disability. *Seizure*, **10**, 401-409.

12

The Role of the Epilepsy Specialist Nurse for People with Learning Disabilities

HEATHER GREGORY

The Grovehill Centre, Beverley, Yorkshire, UK

INTRODUCTION

It is recognised that epilepsy is the most frequently occurring co-morbid condition in people with learning disabilities. As a consequence of this additional handicap their epilepsy is likely to be complex and will often involve more than one seizure type. Their difficulties are further complicated by the presence of increased general health problems, sensory impairments, challenging behaviour, physical disabilities and mental health problems. Furthermore, this group often experiences a range of communication difficulties.

One cannot loose sight of the fact that people with learning disabilities have either *'incomplete or arrested development of mind'* (Mental Health Act, 1983). We must therefore accept and acknowledge that we are dealing with a group of people who have abnormal brain structures or a genetic predisposition to epileptic activity.

The epilepsy of people with learning disability is notoriously difficult to treat effectively and specialist skills are required of all service providers to ensure maximum health gain is achieved.

As the learning disability nurse is specifically trained in the field of learning disability, it would seem pertinent to utilise their core skills and experience by enabling them to develop epilepsy knowledge to a high standard. The learning disability epilepsy nurse is well placed to act as case co-ordinator encompassing both health and social care issues.

THE LEARNING DISABILITY EPILEPSY NURSE

The government has acknowledged the concept of specialist nurses in The New NHS (1997):

'The government is particularly keen to extend developments in the role of nurses working in acute and community services....taking on leadership roles, monitoring and educating nurses and other staff, managing care, developing nurse-led clinics and district-wide services....across organisational and professional boundaries ensuring continuity and integration of care'.

Supporting this specialist role, Hannah and Brodie (1998) suggest that it is the learning disability epilepsy nurse who provides the cohesive link between the person with a learning disability and epilepsy and everyone providing care. They view the learning disability epilepsy nurse as an increasing asset both within the community and the hospital setting due to their dual qualification and training.

A plethora of documents exist to guide professionals in developing epilepsy services, but in order to maximise and extend these theories into the field of learning disability there needs to be an experienced practitioner driving the development of clinical services. Epilepsy services for this group should be based on the general model described in the document *Specification for Epilepsy Services.* They should reflect the aims for people with epilepsy alone, i.e. achieving maximum health gain, reducing morbidity and preventing avoidable death, increased quality of life adjusted years and more effective, efficient use of resources.

However, one needs to consider carefully the specific needs of this population. *Signpost for Success in Commissioning and Providing Health Services For People with Learning Disabilities* (1998) highlights, firstly, that epilepsy is a wider problem than having seizures, and services should focus on quality of life issues; secondly, that treatment is long-term and information, counselling and careful monitoring are required.

This document recommends:

- development of a specialist service that can meet the needs of people with learning disabilities;

- advice and training for people with epilepsy and their carers;

- diagnostic services that can respond to people with special needs (such as the availability of brain scans under anaesthetic);

- close liaison between primary and specialist services.

Some of these recommendations are reflected in recent *Clinical Guidelines for the Management of Epilepsy in Adults with an Intellectual Disability* developed by The Working Group of the International Association of the

Scientific Study of Intellectual Disability (2001). The Standards for Services advocated by this working group recommend that:

- both the medical and psychological impact of epilepsy are assessed adequately, and reviewed regularly;

- carers and staff working with the individual should receive training in epilepsy and its management, and on the impact it has on people's lives;

- training should also be provided on methods of behavioural observation and seizure reporting;

- carers should also be trained in any necessary emergency procedures, such as the rectal administration of medication and resuscitation, and clear policies should be provided for these on an individual basis;

- care plans should ensure consistency in the support offered to people with intellectual disability and epilepsy. For example, the same individual should accompany the person with epilepsy to clinic appointments;

- Accurate records should be kept, using diaries or equivalents, and those working with the person with epilepsy should be familiar with their use.

Nurses can potentially be the most valuable assets in co-ordinating epilepsy care for this group. They are likely to have more direct care contact and thus are able to contribute vital information for individual care plans and provide the key link between primary and secondary care. They are also seen as well placed to give information, support and advice to those with epilepsy, their relatives and carers. Furthermore, they are ideally situated to audit epilepsy services and contribute to maximising local service provision.

The role of the learning disability epilepsy nurse would seem to be multi-faceted. This role can be defined in two main areas, namely general aims and specific components, as shown in Box 1 and Box 2.

Box 1

Learning Disability Epilepsy Nurse.

General Aims of the Role

- Achieving maximum health gain.

- Reducing morbidity and preventing avoidable death.

- Increasing quality of life adjusted years.

- Promoting effective and efficient use of resources.

Box 2

Learning Disability Epilepsy Nurse.

Specific Components of the Role

- Completing epilepsy assessments

- Determining the correct diagnosis of epilepsy and assisting in the detailed investigation of differential diagnosis.

- Defining the type of seizure.

- Providing support and advice to clients and carers through complex medication titration regimes.

- Investigating difficulties in compliance issues related to swallowing difficulties, metabolism, etc.

- Identifying health problems and physical difficulties which affect behaviour and epilepsy.

- Ensuring appropriate treatment, including correct dose and administration of medication.

- Ensuring appropriate monitoring of seizures, including type, frequency and intensity.

- Advising on simple measures to reduce seizures through management of 'triggers'.

- Providing education and information to people with epilepsy, families and professional carers.

- Liaising between health professionals at primary, secondary and tertiary levels.

- Participating in clinical reviews.

- Facilitating nurse led epilepsy clinics.

- Co-ordinating local learning disability specific neurology clinics.

- Developing a database of people with learning disabilities and epilepsy for epidemiological research and audit purposes.

- Auditing developing epilepsy services for people with learning disabilities.

- Evaluating quality of life and other clinical outcomes.

LEARNING DISABILITY EPILEPSY ASSESSMENT

It would seem essential that people with learning disability that have suspected or proven epilepsy be referred to specialist services for a review. The learning disability epilepsy nurse is involved in this process from the onset; they encompass a wide range of essential skills and knowledge of epilepsy and learning disability. The role at this stage is to act as a 'case co-ordinator' to source, collate and consolidate information from a wide range of material. The nurse is in a key position to gather this information from families, resource centres, respite and group homes, schools and colleges, together with a detailed medical and psychiatric history.

In 1988 the author developed an epilepsy assessment specific to people with learning disabilities in response to the particular needs of people with learning disabilities and epilepsy, and in recognition of the difficulties in gathering extensive information from people with communication, comprehension and articulation difficulties. This also evolved to encompass some of the recommendations of a clinical audit study undertaken locally entitled *The Management of Epilepsy for people with a Learning Disability in East Yorkshire.*

Amongst a number of issues, the audit highlighted that:

• assessment of seizures in this group needs specialist consideration;

• for a significant number of people:
  • their medication caused side effects,
  • their epilepsy was unstable,
  • their medication was not reviewed;

• a proportion of people who experienced regular seizures was not seen by specialist services;

• there was insufficient recorded information on frequency and type of seizures.

This Initial Learning Disability Epilepsy Nursing Assessment cited in *Managing Epilepsy* by Taylor (2001) provided an essential tool with which to collate information regarding the person's epilepsy. The initial format and content of this assessment method has evolved through further clinical audit studies and now provides an essential component on which to base a treatment plan. The assessment and guidelines encompass the following information:

• basic client information and contact details of GP, consultants etc.;

• onset of epilepsy and any identified causes;

- descriptions of seizures, including types, frequency, onset, and triggers;
- details of non-epileptic seizures;
- nature of learning disability;
- associated physical or medical problems;
- behavioural problems;
- recording of seizures;
- medication, including current anticonvulsants and any other medication, dose, side effects, preparation and administration, previous medication and reasons for discontinuing medication;
- results of investigations, including neurophysiololgy and/or medical investigations;
- carers' needs;
- clients' needs;
- quality of life issues;
- management of prolonged seizure activity.

This information will be shared with the individual, the carer, the consultant and the general practitioner. Through liaising between primary and secondary care, the learning disability epilepsy nurse enables a seamless delivery of care. Information given by the consultant can also be reinforced and disseminated to all care providers.

In addition to the Epilepsy Nursing Assessment, management plans are also essential to enable bespoke emergency plans to be developed for clients in the event of prolonged seizures or clusters of seizures.

Special consideration needs to be given when developing protocols for the administration of 'rescue medication'. Frequently benzodiazepines are prescribed as standard practice for those whose seizures are not always self - limiting. This can create conflict due to the constraints of social care situations, such as day services or respite services, due to the carer's inability to carry out any care procedure deemed by their policy to be 'invasive'. We must recognise that many carers also feel uneasy at the thought of carrying out a procedure which they perceive to be medical. Through a collaborative approach, the learning disability epilepsy nurse should establish a clear, concise, individual management plan which recognises these limitations. Carers need to know when, what and how to administer these medications.

Often care is received from a wide range of service providers where continuity of treatment is essential. Here the individual Epilepsy Management Plan can provide essential information for the service provider about what to do in the emergency situation or how to manage and prevent clusters of seizures. Through careful monitoring, the effectiveness of managing seizures in this manner can be established. The learning disability epilepsy nurse is really in a key position to collate all available information.

DIFFERENTIAL DIAGNOSIS

The combination of learning disability and epilepsy, together with communication difficulties and additional health needs, can cause considerable problems of diagnosis, as well as confusing accurate seizure monitoring and appropriate treatment. It is recognised that people with learning disabilities often present with several different seizure types, which are commonly refractory to treatment. In addition, correct diagnosis can be complicated through the difficulties of differential diagnosis.

Syncope, non-epileptic attack disorder, psychosis and sleep apnoea may be mistaken for seizures. These differential diagnoses occur both in the general population with epilepsy and in people with learning disabilities who have epilepsy. However, they are less likely to be recognised in the latter group. Moreover, it can be immensely difficult to differentiate between epilepsy-induced abnormal behaviours with environmentally-influenced behaviours and partial epilepsy in someone who routinely presents with unusual movement disorders. The accuracy of classification is limited by communication abilities: the prevalence of partial seizures may be underestimated due partly to carers' inability to recognise these subtle seizures; communication difficulties may make the recognition of aura and post-ictal phenomena difficult.

The process of diagnosing epilepsy relies in part on an eyewitness account of the episode. However, diagnostic overshadowing complicates differentiating between seizures and disturbances of behaviour. An expectation for the episode to be either epilepsy or a behaviour problem can influence the description of the episode. Routine and ambulatory electroencephalograms with telemetry are helpful to differentiate between seizure activity and behavioural disorders, but people with learning disabilities may refuse to have a waking EEG.

The learning disability epilepsy nurse is able to facilitate a co-ordinated approach to aid the correct diagnosis of epilepsy. Accurate history taking and careful consideration of the medical history (detailed perusal of medical and psychiatric notes) can often help identify the initial diagnosis. The specialist nurse can help prevent abortive attempts at investigations by providing meaningful advice and information about EEGs, Computerised Tomography and MRI. Through regular liaison with these specialist departments, the specialist nurse can provide a valuable link between technicians and the person with learning disabilities, thus enabling a cohesive approach, minimising the anxieties that may arise for the individual.

A number of adults with epilepsy and learning disability may not have had their epilepsy reviewed by neurology services. For this population, it is essential that a detailed evaluation of all clinical information relating to the diagnosis of their epilepsy be reviewed. People may have been mistakenly diagnosed with epilepsy following one seizure event, and may have remained on high doses of mixed polypharmacy unnecessarily. Conversely, people with frontal or temporal lobe epilepsy may have been inappropriately treated with tranquillisers or antipsychotic medication, and may have been mismanaged, as their complex partial seizures have not been identified or have been misdiagnosed. Historically, due to the inherent difficulties in identifying frontal and temporal lobe seizures, these people may not have been referred to neurology or psychiatry for review of their epilepsy as their generalised seizures, which are easily identifiable, may have been controlled. The learning disability epilepsy nurse needs to ensure that carers and colleagues are fully aware of the possibility of these complex partial seizures occurring through epilepsy awareness training.

PHYSICAL AND OTHER HEALTH PROBLEMS AFFECTING EPILEPSY

The health surveillance of people with learning disabilities is frequently sadly neglected, yet this population often has increasing healthcare needs. Compared to the comprehensive screening for cervical, breast and testicular cancers and hypertension, this population is inadequately supported. Furthermore, up to one third of people with learning disabilities have an associated physical disability, usually cerebral palsy. The problems associated with unidentified increased health care needs and physical disabilities further compound the dual diagnosis of epilepsy and learning disabilities. The learning disability epilepsy nurse can co-ordinate a multi-disciplinary assessment involving, for example, speech and language therapists, dieticians and neurologists, to identify the most appropriate treatment regimens and management.

There is anecdotal evidence to suggest that alternative feeding and medication routes such as per-cutaneous gastrostomy can significantly improve seizure control. Nutritional problems and constipation can affect behaviour and can make epilepsy worse. It is necessary to identify a means of managing these often chronic problems in order to prevent seizures occurring. The learning disability epilepsy nurse, together with the physiotherapist and dietician, can assess the specific needs of the individual and develop a relevant care plan. Recent research by Emly *et al.* (2002) acknowledges the benefits of abdominal massage for this group as an effective means of managing chronic constipation, reducing the need for long-term laxatives. Other health-related problems include infections of the urinary and upper respiratory tracts, which are often insidious, worsening behaviour and epilepsy. It is often difficult for the carer to identify these infections and the first sign may be onset of seizure activity. Learning disability nurses are becoming increasingly aware of the necessity to assess the healthcare needs of people with learning disabilities beyond any epilepsy. Providing regular health screening, health education and identifying methods of preventing and managing health related problems could lead to more effective means of managing a person's epilepsy.

In many respects, the effective care pathway for epilepsy services can provide a template for improving access and provision of equitable health care across all disciplines for both primary and secondary care providers. *Valuing People* (2001) suggests Health Action Plans as the answer to co-ordinated effective health care for people with learning disabilities in many areas, and epilepsy care for this client group is providing the gold standard.

PERSON CENTRED PLANNING

In 1972 Wolfensberger developed the philosophy of 'Normalisation', focusing on the rights of people with learning disabilities. People were to be perceived as 'people first' and 'disability second' and more value was placed on the individual being the focal point when considering service delivery. These initial philosophies were later expanded by O'Brien (1987) and Sanderson (1987) who considered the choices of individuals and the need to explore their own experiences and perspectives. In 2001 the White Paper *Valuing People* was launched, which highlighted these theories further in the thrust to develop services for people with learning disabilities through 'Person Centred Planning'.

'Person centred planning is a process for continual listening and learning, focussed on what is important to someone now and for the future, and acting upon this alliance with the family and friends.' (Valuing People, DOH 2001)

The principles of Person Centred Planning should be at the root of all service developments, not least in the development of epilepsy services and the methods used to support families.

In terms of epilepsy, this would include enabling the individual to consider how their epilepsy affects their life and to utilise creative and imaginative methods in providing information on all aspects of epilepsy, as outlined in the section on *Developing and Designing Information on Epilepsy Services*. This would empower individuals and enable them to make choices. Their priorities can be reflected in a bespoke treatment plan. It is also important to consider the needs of the family and carers supporting the service user; family and carer issues are explored in the section entitled *Working with Carers.*

The learning disability epilepsy nurse can enable individuals to become more involved with the management of their epilepsy by adopting approaches that include them. Some of these approaches have been discussed previously and would include the following areas:

• designing information specifically for the service user;

• developing courses on epilepsy for the service user;

• enabling the individual to monitor and record their seizures by designing individual recording systems;

• encouraging self-administration of medication, through use of nomad systems and careful supervision;

• including the service user when developing individual Epilepsy Management Plans;

• empowering the service user and the families;

• including the service user in the development of individual risk assessment;

As Oona Cunningham (2000) suggests:

> *'We should place clients at the centre of care planning, give them 'owner-ship' of their epilepsy and create a collective approach in minimising the impact the epilepsy has on their quality of life. We should foster the growing momentum away from practices that exclude clients and their perspective and develop methods that forge alliances and inclusive frame-works.'*

Other issues to consider are *Risk Management* and *Consent.*

Risk Management

The ethos of risk management should be to minimise the risk for the individual and those caring for them, but often this has developed into strategies to protect organisations from risk of litigation. The issues of risk management are wholly individual, so Person Centred Planning should be employed as the means to develop an effective Risk Management Plan that balances safety with quality of life.

Issues that may arise could be:

• overprotection;

- high levels of supervision;

- inability to object to risk management methods in some situations;

- risk management can either potentially improve safety or restrict life opportunities.

Consent

When entering into any treatment plan, it is essential to ensure that the client gives informed consent if there is the capacity to do so. If there is lack of capacity, it is important to be able to demonstrate that any treatment offered is in that person's interests (Department of Health, 2001). Surgeons are understandably keen to have consent forms signed before any procedure, but there has historically been less emphasis placed upon medical intervention. The concept of implied consent, that is opening the mouth to take medication, would seem appropriate in those who are aware that they are receiving medication and why. Many of us feel less comfortable with regard to those who are simply compliant without understanding.

The administration of medication covertly in food or drink would be seen as unlawful, as in a person who has the capacity to give or withhold consent and chooses to refuse treatment. In someone unable to give consent, this practice must be demonstrably in their best interests (UKCC, 2001). A useful system for both establishing the capacity of a person with learning disability to give informed consent, and providing a framework for ensuring clinical interventions are in someone's best interests if unable to consent, has been put forward by Constable (2001).

DEVELOPING AND DESIGNING
INFORMATION ON EPILEPSY AND SERVICES

The individual's ability to manage and cope with their epilepsy may be influenced through their knowledge and understanding of their condition. The learning disability epilepsy nurse can play a key role in identifying methods of communicating and creating information that is meaningful for service users. This could be done in collaboration with speech and language therapy colleagues. Information packs illustrating the local epilepsy services available from neurology or psychiatry departments can be developed to include photographs of these departments and the process of assessment and investigation. These packs could also illustrate the neurophysiology department and the process of investigations, together with contact details for local services available to support the service user.

Medication information sheets could be modified and can include symbols to illustrate possible side effects and so on. The organisation Mencap has produced a useful guide for accessible writing entitled *Am I making myself clear?* (Mencap 2000), which highlights the importance of utilising photographs, signs and symbols to support the written word. It also recognises the value of audio and videotapes to overcome the difficulties of disseminating complex information in a meaningful way. Video recordings of seizures can help people to understand the various seizure types and practical ways of managing seizures.

The series *Books Beyond Words* include a book entitled *Getting on with Epilepsy* (Hollins, Bernal and Thacker, 1999) designed specifically for individuals unable to read. This resource would seem particularly useful when exploring service user's feelings about their epilepsy. Many have had their condition for many years and may not have had the opportunity to discuss their personal fears and beliefs about their epilepsy. They may have developed inappropriate preconceived ideas about restricting their lifestyle because of their epilepsy. Or conversely, they may be at risk of inducing seizures through lack of knowledge of triggers. Lifestyle issues need to be explored with service users in a meaningful way to develop support systems which will promote life experiences through careful risk management. Other resources specifically designed for people with moderate learning disabilities have recently been published by the National Society for Epilepsy and Epilepsy Action.

A study undertaken by Clarke *et al.* (2001), which evaluated a video-assisted educational pack for adults with mild learning disabilities and epilepsy entitled *Epilepsy and You* (Paul, 1996), found this package to be suitable for a wide range of individuals and demonstrated significant gains in knowledge. Their results suggest that, although adults with epilepsy and mild learning disability may know how epilepsy presents in behavioural terms, they were not likely to understand the physiological mechanisms behind epilepsy or appreciate seizure recording. Furthermore, they found that whilst knowledge about medication was not poor, there were deficits in knowledge regarding: why it was important to visit doctors; what an EEG is; and how medication works. In addition, they also found that, whilst some individuals had some knowledge about safety issues, there was little known about the use and importance of seizure diaries. The results from the study not only indicated that individuals enjoyed taking part in the training, but also suggested that the training offered individuals more control over their health, encouraged medication compliance, and may therefore minimise secondary psychological consequences of epilepsy.

The epilepsy specialist nurse can collate and develop a wide range of resources relating to epilepsy, assisting the person with a learning disability to gain greater understanding about their condition and about the necessity for various investigative techniques and treatment options. This acquired knowledge will empower the individual thus enabling them to make informed choices and contribute to the effective management of their epilepsy. Furthermore, it will promote a greater awareness of the management of seizure 'triggers' and risk management.

WORKING WITH CARERS

People with learning disabilities live in a variety of different care settings. Their carers include private and voluntary agencies, Social Services, parents, elderly carers and siblings.

Whilst Social Services, private agencies and the voluntary sector are service providers for some people with learning disabilities and epilepsy, it is recognised that the majority of people with learning disability are cared for by family carers (Ward, 2000). This section will therefore focus mainly on working with families and will consider: the impact of caring, opportunities to 'empower carers', and the conflict that can exist between carers and professionals.

Family Matters (Ward, 2000), a project commissioned by the Department of Health to develop the New Learning Disability Strategy, considered the views of families who care for people with learning disabilities. This document suggests that 'Care in the Community is Family Care' and that families provide the main support for men and women with learning disabilities in the United Kingdom. Furthermore, carers are perceived to be pivotal in maintaining people with learning disabilities in the community. The document highlights that 60% of adults live with families and one third of these live with a carer over 70 years old. Carer organisations estimate there are six million carers in the UK, saving the public purse £34 billion pounds (Princess Royal Trust for Carers, 1998).

In some services a culture has developed that perceives families as a problem and difficult to work with. Families can be seen as the barrier to enabling their relative to gain greater independence, yet this misperception can oversimplify complex family relationships and the real contribution that families make throughout their relatives' lives. Families who care for people with the dual diagnosis of epilepsy and learning disability face the enormous day-to-day challenge of managing the complex care issues involved in supporting their relative. Services need to find constructive ways to work with families in the best interests of people with epilepsy and learning disabilities. The learning disability epilepsy nurse needs to fully appreciate the impact of caring and offer as much information, advice and support as possible to the families and other relatives with this dual diagnosis. Carers need to feel that their role in minimising the effects of the epilepsy and thus promoting independence and health gain benefits not only their relative, but also the whole family.

When working with families of people with learning disabilities and epilepsy, the learning disability epilepsy nurse needs to appreciate the unique circumstances of each individual family. There is no such thing as a typical person with learning disabilities and epilepsy; all are unique, in the same way as families are all unique. Their needs are diverse and complex, but, in addition, the caring role for families is often life long. Carers may also have taken the role of multiple carers, not only caring for their son/daughter with learning disability and epilepsy, but also caring for ageing and frail grandparents, and for grandchildren, as the necessity of being at home enables them to take on this multiple caring role.

There are particular caring issues for elderly carers. They continue to care but are getting older and in need of more social and healthcare themselves. They are likely to have reduced social networks as spouse or family die and their relationship with their son/daughter may develop into one of mutual dependency. They may believe that if they are seen not to be coping, their son or daughter could be taken into care. But often the reality is that Social Services would be unable to provide an adequate care alternative.

Seizure reduction may also have an implication on benefits and the loss of the caring role. Elderly carers may be resistant to the positive effects of newer medication, as it reduces their ability to care. Some of the newer anticonvulsants with fewer side effects have replaced older anticonvulsant drugs and may release their relative from a state of sedation to a state of relative alertness. The learning disability epilepsy nurse needs to work closely with families in order to raise awareness of this possibility, since it may result in carers being unable to continue caring.

Furthermore, one needs to examine and appreciate the impact of belief systems, attitudes, social and cultural diversities, personalities, financial and social standing, as all these factors can influence the outcome of any epilepsy management plan. Unravelling all these complex influences can be difficult and time consuming, yet is extremely important in the learning disability epilepsy nurse's role to facilitate a process which encompasses mutual trust and respect for each person's contribution in the treatment process.

In examining the impact of the caring role, Mencap (2000) interviewed 76 families caring for people with profound multiple disabilities including epilepsy and learning disability. The document identified that:

- 60% of families cared for more than 18 hours a day (10 hours on basic physical care);

- carers received an average of 20 minutes support from social services a day;

- carers were woken an average of three times a night;

- one third of carers had a continuous caring role.

It may seem inconceivable that, with the shift to 'Community Care', family carers continue to provide this amount of care. However, the complex intractable nature of this dual diagnosis together with the additional health-care needs of this group, often challenge the services designed to meet their needs. Where services fail to meet such complex needs, it is the family carers who are left with the ongoing burden.

People with learning disability and epilepsy may be returned home from local authority day centres due to seizure activity, or excluded from services due to the severity of their epilepsy causing unsettled behaviour. Often it is the service policies and cultures that induce stress in carers, as Williams and Robinson (2000) highlight:

'Stress is caused more often with the service system than by any particular characteristics of the person with a learning disability.'

Attendance at specialist epilepsy clinics can be stressful, due to distance of the acute hospitals, poor disabled facilities, little support in waiting areas, long waiting times at clinics, difficulties in understanding complex information relating to seizures, investigations or treatment changes. Furthermore, where the person has complex health needs in addition to their epilepsy and learning disability, different specialists may review them.

The author is aware of one family caring for two sons with profound learning and physical disabilities who had 32 outpatient appointments in one year. The role of the learning disability epilepsy nurse was to co-ordinate a multi-specialist approach that rationalised a more systematic provision of treatment and review, thus reducing the number of outpatient appointments.

The effects of caring may induce high levels of stress, influence the families finances (people surrender their careers to care), induce isolation, affect relationships with friends and relatives and can lead to marital breakdown. The role of the learning disability epilepsy nurse is to recognise these effects of caring, liaise with support services to provide counselling and support to relatives, but moreover to be continually aware of the additional stress that may result from any treatment changes relating to the relative's epilepsy.

Families may need additional support to identify seizure activity. However, a simple request to observe and record seizure activity may actually add to the already complex stressful role of caring.

Families who care for people with complex epilepsy and learning disability seem to appreciate direct support given at home from experienced health-care staff. The learning disability epilepsy nurse can enlist this support through targeting funds from 'Direct Payments', 'Independent Living Fund' and/or 'Continuing Healthcare Monies', whichever is the most appropriate locally. These experienced healthcare staff can support the person with learning disability and epilepsy, assist in the identification of seizure activity, monitor and record seizure activity, and provide emotional and respite support to the family.

Person Centred Planning, as mentioned previously, can help focus on the needs of the individual, and is a process that will engage both professionals and families.

To give a example of this approach, the author was involved in a local clinical audit study examining epilepsy services for people with learning disabilities, which collected information from professionals in primary and secondary services. The audit focused on the relationship between primary and secondary care, and included client's and carer's experiences of epilepsy services, which were collated through a structured questionnaire. The identified needs of families were highlighted in the outcomes of the audit and reflected in the development of local specialist epilepsy services for people with learning disabilities.

Following this audit, the specific needs of families are now met through:

• local community based learning disability specific neurology clinics;

• carers needs included in the Epilepsy Assessment;

• fast track to services;

• disabled Parking and access to clinics;

• reduced waiting time at clinics;

• counselling;

• clear information;

• follow-up epilepsy nursing support;

• support to manage change.

EPILEPSY AWARENESS TRAINING

Families need information and training in epilepsy. Provision of epilepsy awareness enables them to understand and value the contribution new treatments can make to someone's epilepsy. They will be able to recognise different seizures and understand the causes of epilepsy and triggers of seizures. Awareness of how drugs work and how to administer them improves compliance and seizure control. Epilepsy Awareness Training is one of the crucial factors involved in enabling carers to feel confident about their relative's epilepsy. The learning disability epilepsy nurse is in a key position through experience and dual training in learning disability and epilepsy to design and facilitate epilepsy awareness training for carers. Through this information, carers can effect positive influences on their relative's treatment plan and work more closely in partnership with professionals. As Gibran states:

'If he is indeed wise he does not bid you enter the house of his wisdom, but rather leads you to the threshold of your own mind.' (Kahil Gibran, *The Prophet*)

Where organisations place the value of the individual with a learning disability and epilepsy at the core of an organisational structure, this will be reflected in the value of the support staff employed to provide management. A poor value base is often reflected in staff shortages, sickness, inadequate training, poor pay and conditions. The learning disability epilepsy nurse can support these organisations through provision of Epilepsy Awareness Training for their staff, and include staff in developing epilepsy management plans, risk assessments and care plans.

The role of the learning disability epilepsy nurse includes facilitating Epilepsy Awareness Training for paid carers and families and people with learning disabilities and epilepsy. The knowledge base and experience of the nurse ensure meeting the key objectives of this training. The epilepsy training programme should be designed to be flexible and adaptable in meeting the needs of different service providers, families and people with learning disabilities. The complex information involved in epilepsy needs to be assimilated in a way that can be easily understood and maintained. Training groups of staff is an economical use of nursing time, as it can improve the information gathered by carers, improve recording of seizures, promote good understanding amongst care staff and improve the standard of care given, all of which reduce the clinical input needed over time.

Depending on the target group, the learning disability epilepsy nurse can be selective regarding the content and depth of the training session. Whilst the following list of topic headings is by no means exhaustive, it attempts to include the relevant subjects that could be included in a Learning Disability Epilepsy Awareness Programme

- The History of Epilepsy

- Epidemiology

- Diagnosis

- Differential Diagnosis

- Investigations

- Specific Epileptic Syndromes

- Treatment (including medication, surgery, complementary therapies)

- Triggers of seizures

- Recording Methods

- Seizure Management

- Administration of Emergency Treatments
- Preparing for Neurology Clinic

CLINICAL AUDIT

One could suggest that the key to developing meaningful epilepsy services for this group is the utilisation of the clinical audit process. NICE (2000) suggest that clinical audit is at the heart of clinical governance as it:

- provides the mechanisms for reviewing the quality of everyday care provided to patients;
- addresses quality issues systematically and explicitly providing reliable information;
- can confirm the quality of clinical services and highlight the need for improvement.

This systematic approach in reviewing and developing services would seem to provide one of the most effective means of assessing the need for services and developing frameworks in which to build future services. With the knowledge and experience of learning disability, epilepsy, service providers and the local area, the learning disability epilepsy nurse is in a key central position to facilitate the clinical audit process. The author, as an epilepsy learning disability nurse, has facilitated three clinical audit studies considering epilepsy services for people with learning disabilities and epilepsy. The audit process has proved to be an effective tool in evaluating and reviewing current management of epilepsy services, and this evaluative process has enabled epilepsy services to develop based on specific needs within the local community healthcare trust. In particular, it has provided a format to include the views of people with epilepsy, families, carers and service providers including GPs, consultant neurologists, neurophysiologists, community learning disability nurses and epilepsy nurses. The recommendations of the audit studies have provided a framework in which to design and develop locally based services on the specific needs of the group whilst maximising the use of local resources. They have also enabled the nurse as a service developer together with colleagues to highlight to service managers where resources could be utilised in the local area and advise on service developments.

It is recognised that the management of epilepsy in people with learning disability is complex. The issues for this group are often sadly neglected and rarely featured as a priority agenda on local hospital and community health care trusts service development agendas. The learning disability epilepsy specialist nurse, through clinical audit processes, can shift the focus and highlight the chronic complex needs of this group and contribute to the development of meaningful services through the creative utilisation of existing resources and the expansion of local services.

CONCLUSION

The introduction of specialist epilepsy nurses has progressed the care of people with epilepsy over recent years. The recognition that people with learning disabilities would benefit from the intervention of nurses from the field of learning disability with specific training in epilepsy has led to an overwhelming improvement in care standards and quality of life.

The role of the learning disability epilepsy nurse has developed to enable this group with such complex needs to receive the range of specialist diagnostic and treatment services available today for people with epilepsy. Those involved in this therapeutic pathway are not just health professionals but also families, carers, social services, employment and educational agencies, and private sector and voluntary agencies. The learning disability epilepsy nurse is in a key position to coordinate epilepsy services for this group.

REFERENCES

Clarke, A.J., Espie, C.A. and Paul, A. (2001). Adults with learning disabilities and epilepsy: knowledge about epilepsy before and after an educational package. *Seizure* **10**, 492-499.

Constable. M. (2001). Adults with learning disability, how can healthcare professional ensure best practice in relation to examination and treatment. *The Journal of the Association of Practitioners in Learning Disabilities* **17**, 7-11.

Cunningham, O. (2000). Person Centred Planning. *Learning Disability Practice* **3**, 16–19.

Department of Health (1993). *Mental Health Act 1983*. HMSO, London.

Department of Health (1997). *The New NHS*. HMSO, London.

Department of Health (1998). *Signposts for Success in Commissioning and Providing Health Services for People with Learning Disabilities*. HMSO, London.

Department of Health (2001). *Reference Guide to Consent for Examination and Treatment*. HMSO, London.

Department of Health (2001). *Valuing People: A new strategy for Learning Disability for the 21st Century*. HMSO, London.

Emly, M. *et al.* (2002). Abdominal massage for adults with learning disabilities. *Nursing Times* **57**, 63.

Hannah, J.A. and Brodie, M.J. (1998). Epilepsy and learning disabilities – a challenge for the next millennium? *Seizure* **7**, 3-13.

Hollins, S., Bernal, J. and Thacker, A. (1999). *Getting on with Epilepsy*. Books Beyond Words, Gaskell, London.

Mencap (2000). *Am I Making Myself Clear? Mencap's Guidelines for Accessible Writing*. Mencap.

Mencap (2002). No ordinary life. *Learning Disability Practice* **5**, 8-9.

NICE (2000). *Principles for Best Practice in Clinical Audit.* Radcliffe Medical Press, Oxford.

O'Brien, A. (1987). A guide to lifestyle planning. In: Wilcox, B. and Bellamy, T. (Eds), *A Comprehensive Guide to Activities Catalogue.* Paul Brookes Publishing, Baltimore.

Paul, A. (1996). *Epilepsy and You.* Pavillion Publishing, Brighton.

Princess Royal Trust For Carers (1998). *Eight Hours a Day and Taken for Granted.* Princess Royal Trust for Carers, London.

Sanderson, H. (1987). Essential lifestyle planning. *Focus* **19**, 12-17.

UCB Pharma. Ltd. (2003). Learning Disability and Epilepsy. *Learning Disability Nurse Educational Resource.* UCB Pharma Ltd, Watford.

UKCC (2001). *UKCC Position Statement on the Covert Administration of Medicines. HMSO,* London.

Ward, C.(2000). *Family Matters.* Department of Health, London.

Williams, C. and Robinson, V. (2000). *In Their Own Right: One Year On.* Norah Fry Centre, Bristol.

Wolfensberger, W. W. (1972). *The Principle of Normalisation in Human Services.* National Institute on Mental Retardation, Toronto.

Working Group of the International Association of the Scientific Study of Intellectual Disability. (2001). Clinical guidelines for the management of epilepsy in adults with an intellectual disability. *Seizure* **10**, 401-409.

Youssef, H.A. and Waddington, J.L. (1988). Involuntary orofacial movements in hospitalised patients with mental handicap or epilepsy: relationship to developmental/intellectual deficit and presence or absence of long-term exposure to neuroleptics. *J Neurol Neurosurg Psychiatry* **51**, 863-865.

Index

Page numbers in *italics* refer to figures and tables.